ENDOCRINOLOGY RESEARCH AND CLINICAL DEVELOPMENTS

THE PITUITARY GLAND AND ADRENAL GLANDS

NEW RESEARCH

ENDOCRINOLOGY RESEARCH AND CLINICAL DEVELOPMENTS

THE PITUITARY GLAND AND ADRENAL GLANDS

NEW RESEARCH

NOÉMI BARTA
EDITOR

Medicine & Health
New York

Library of Congress Cataloging-in-Publication Data

ISBN: 978-1-53617-605-6

Published by Nova Science Publishers, Inc. † New York

CONTENTS

PREFACE

In *The Pituitary Gland and Adrenal Glands: New Research*, the authors first discuss pituicytomas, rare primary glial neoplasms that arise in the neurohypophysis (or posterior portion) of the pituitary gland. They typically present with signs and symptoms of a slow growing, non-hormonally active mass of the sellar and suprasellar region, compressing adjacent structures.

Following this, the clinical and pathologic features of spindle cell oncocytomas are discussed. Spindle cell oncocytomas are rare tumors, accounting for less than 0.5% of sellar masses. Tumors typically present in adults and most commonly manifest with visual disturbances and pituitary hypofunction.

Additionally, the authors review the clinical and pathological features of gangliocytomas, rare benign tumors of the neuroaxis. They are most commonly seen in children and young adults, and most often arise in the cerebellum as part of Cowden's disease, or in the sellar region.

The clinicopathologic features of granular tumors, rare neoplasms that most commonly arise in the neurohypophysis or posterior portion of the pituitary gland, are also discussed.

This compilation goes on to examine the adrenal glands, paired structures located superior to the kidneys in the retroperitoneal space. Mineralocorticoids, glucocorticoids and adrenal androgens are synthesized respectively in the zona glomerulosa, zona fasciculatis and zona reticularis that make up the cortex, while the inner adrenal medulla produces the catecholamines and peptides.

The risk of developing adrenal insufficiency among glucocorticoid users is assessed, and risk factors are identified. Glucocorticoids are widely used for the treatment of various inflammatory conditions and malignancies, as well as after organ transplantation.

The closing study explores hypothalamic-pituitary-adrenal axis activation, a potent and complex response to heat stress in domestic livestock. The hypothalamic-pituitary-adrenal axis is activated during stress, which leads to the secretion of cortisol and aldosterone from the adrenal gland.

Chapter 1 - Pituicytomas are rare primary glial neoplasms that arise in the neurohypophysis, or posterior portion of the pituitary gland. They typically present with signs and symptoms of a slow growing, non-hormonally active mass of the sellar and suprasellar region, compressing adjacent structures. Histologically, they are marked by a proliferation of bipolar spindled cells arranged in fascicles or in a storiform pattern. They lack features of high grade gliomas such as prominent mitotic activity, necrosis and vascular proliferation. They also lack features of other astrocytoma variant tumors including Rosenthal fibers and eosinophilic granular bodies. They stain strongly with antibody to S-100 protein and variably with GFAP antibody. Interestingly, they also have been recently noted to stain with antibody to TTF-1. Ki-67 labeling indices are usually low. In 2007, the World Health Organization formally recognized the tumor in its classification schema and designated it as a grade I neoplasm. Treatment includes surgical resection; incompletely resected tumors may grow back over time. This chapter will review the clinicopathologic features of these tumors and discuss differential diagnostic considerations.

Chapter 2 - In 2002, Roncaroli et al. reported the first 5 cases of a mitochondrial-rich, spindled cell tumor presumably arising in the adenohypophysis of the pituitary gland. They coined the name "spindle cell oncocytoma." For the entity. Spindle cell oncocytomas are rare tumors, accounting for less than 0.5% of sellar masses. Tumors typically present in adults and most commonly manifest with visual disturbances and pituitary hypofunction. On imaging and gross inspection, these tumors may resemble pituitary adenomas. Microscopically, they are marked by interlacing fascicles of spindled cells with eosinophilic cytoplasm. Tumors may demonstrate some degree of nuclear atypia. Cell proliferation rates are low. These tumors do not express neuroendocrine and hormonal immunomarkers typically seen in pituitary adenomas. They do express S-100 protein, EMA and BCL2 immunoreactivity. Similar to pituicytomas and granular cell tumors, they also show evidence of thyroid transcription factor-1 (TTF-1) immunoreactivity, suggesting that these tumors may in fact originate from pituicytes in the neurohypophysis of the gland. Spindle cell oncocytomas are considered to be benign (World Health Organization grade I neoplasms). A subset of tumors have been reported to recur after several years, particularly if incompletely resected. This chapter will review the clinical and pathologic features of these neoplasms.

Chapter 3 - Gangliocytomas are rare benign tumors of the neuroaxis. They most commonly arise in children and young adults and most often arise in the cerebellum as part of Cowden's disease (Lhermitte-Duclos disease) or in the sellar region. Isolated sellar gangliocytomas comprise about 0.3-0.5% of all sellar lesions. A subset of sellar gangliocytomas have been described in association with pituitary adenomas; these mixed tumors comprise about 0.5-1.25% of all sellar region tumors. Most of these combined tumors are associated with endocrinopathies, most commonly acromegaly. Multiple theories have been proposed regarding the histogenesis of these mixed tumors. This chapter will review the clinical and pathologic features of these rare mixed tumors and discuss the proposed theories behind their origin.

Chapter 4 - Granular tumors are relatively rare neoplasms that most commonly arise in the neurohypophysis or posterior portion of the pituitary gland. Most present in adults, with a peak incidence in the 5th and 6th decades of life, and they are more frequently encountered in women. These tumors most commonly present with visual field defects secondary to compression of the optic chiasm. The lesion is typically well circumscribed and lobulated. The lesion is marked by a proliferation of large polygonal or slightly elongated cells which contain abundant granular eosinophilic cytoplasm, as its name suggests. The granular quality of the cytoplasm is due to the large number of phagolysosomes that fill it. Immunophenotypically, granular cell tumors, like pituicytomas and spindle cell oncocytomas, are characterized by strong nuclear staining with antibody to thyroid transcription factor-1, suggesting that the tumor is derived from pituicytes in the neurohypophysis. Granular cell tumors are generally considered benign tumors and surgical resection is the treatment of choice for larger and symptomatic lesions. This chapter will review the clinicopathologic features of this neoplasm and include a discussion of differential diagnosis.

Chapter 5 - The adrenal glands are paired structures located superior to the kidneys in the retroperitoneal space. Mineralocorticoids, glucocorticoids and adrenal androgens are synthesized respectively in the zona glomerulosa, zona fasciculatis and zona reticularisthat make up the cortex, while the inner adrenal medulla produces the catecholamines and peptides. Aldosterone, the main mineralocorticoid, regulates circulating fluid volume and electrolyte balance by promoting sodium and chloride retention by the distal tubule while potassium is excreted. The main active glucocorticoid cortisol generates a catabolic state that characterizes the body's response to stress by increasing blood glucose, stimulating lipolysis and generating anti-inflammatory and immunosuppressive effects.The secretion of adrenal hormones is controlled and regulated by a negative feedback system, called the Hypothalamo-Pituitary-Adrenal Axis. Adrenal insufficiency, as identified by low levels of morning cortisol, can be primary or secondary. Primary adrenal insufficiency is caused by congenital enzymatic defects or tissue destruction from autoimmune etiology while secondary insufficiency is caused by ACTH deficiency.Primary hyperaldosteronism as identified by high aldosterone-renin ratio is a treatable disorder caused mostly by a functional adenoma. Benign functional or nonfunctional adenomas are the most common adrenal tumors while metastases to the adrenals are the most common malignant tumors. Incidentalomas which are detected incidentally may be a cause for subclinical Cushing's syndrome if they are functional.

Exogenous use of excess glucocorticoids may cause Cushing Syndrome which may be lethal if not identified early and treated appropriately. Adrenal surgery can be performed laparoscopically or via an open approach. Laparoscopy can be transabdominal or posterior retroperitoneal. The surgical technique is based on the experience of the surgeon as well as on the patient and tumor characteristics.

Chapter 6 - Glucocorticoids are widely used for the treatment of various inflammatory conditions, malignancies and after organ transplantation. The use of glucocorticoids is associated with numerous side effects. Glucocorticoids are considered the most common cause of tertiary adrenal insufficiency. Therefore, patients may require glucocorticoid replacement therapy after chronic use of glucocorticoids. There are few studies in the published literature that have approached the assessment of the hypothalamo-pituitary-adrenal axis function following glucocorticoid therapy. As a result, there has been little consensus in the components of glucocorticoid exposure (dose and time) that may contribute to the hypothalamo-pituitary-adrenal axis suppression and potential recovery. The general approach in most centers is to gradually taper the dose of glucocorticoids to diminish the risk of adrenal insufficiency following glucocorticoid withdrawal. This chapter is aimed to obtain knowledge about the risk of developing adrenal insufficiency among glucocorticoid users and identify risk factors. Secondary aims are to explore if some features of the hypothalamo-pituitary-adrenal axis function testing could guide physicians to identify those groups of patients at higher risk of presenting with adrenal insufficiency.

Chapter 7 - The rising global temperature has been a major concern in livestock production as it affects the productive performance of livestock across the globe. Heat stress has been proven to be detrimental to the livestock industry and has resulted in huge economic losses due to reduction in production. Domestic animals exhibit various biological response mechanisms to survive the harsh climatic conditions and neuro-endocrine regulation of stress response was considered the primary mechanisms by which the animals survive the stress. The hypothalamic-pituitary-adrenal (HPA) axis activation is a potent and complex response to heat stress in domestic livestock. The HPA axis is activated during stress which leads to the secretion of cortisol and aldosterone, from adrenal gland. The cortisol secreted from adrenal cortex was considered to be the ideal stress marker in livestock. The cortisol which is the primary glucocorticoid released from the adrenal cortex, mainly target liver, muscle and adipose tissue to initiate gluconeogenesis, glycogenolysis, lipolysis and proteolysis mechanisms in stressed animals thereby restoring their energy homeostasis while aldosterone maintains the electrolyte balance in them. The release of these steroid hormones plays a vital role to ameliorate heat stress in farm animals. Being the prime sensor of stress, the adrenal gland plays a significant role in maintaining homeostasis and thereby reducing the detrimental effects of heat stress in livestock.

In: The Pituitary Gland and Adrenal Glands
Editor: Noémi Barta
ISBN: 978-1-53617-605-6

Chapter 1

PITUITCYTOMA: A CLINICOPATHOLOGIC REVIEW OF A RARE GLIAL NEOPLASM OF THE PITUITARY

John L. McAfee, BA and Richard A. Prayson*, MD, MEd
Cleveland Clinic Lerner College of Medicine and Department of Anatomic Pathology, Cleveland Clinic
Cleveland, Ohio

ABSTRACT

Pituicytomas are rare primary glial neoplasms that arise in the neurohypophysis, or posterior portion of the pituitary gland. They typically present with signs and symptoms of a slow growing, non-hormonally active mass of the sellar and suprasellar region, compressing adjacent structures. Histologically, they are marked by a proliferation of bipolar spindled cells arranged in fascicles or in a storiform pattern. They lack features of high grade gliomas such as prominent mitotic activity, necrosis and vascular proliferation. They also lack features of other astrocytoma variant tumors including Rosenthal fibers and eosinophilic

* Corresponding Author's E-mail: praysor@ccf.org.

granular bodies. They stain strongly with antibody to S-100 protein and variably with GFAP antibody. Interestingly, they also have been recently noted to stain with antibody to TTF-1. Ki-67 labeling indices are usually low. In 2007, the World Health Organization formally recognized the tumor in its classification schema and designated it as a grade I neoplasm. Treatment includes surgical resection; incompletely resected tumors may grow back over time. This chapter will review the clinicopathologic features of these tumors and discuss differential diagnostic considerations.

INTRODUCTION

Pituicytomas are rare neoplasms of the sellar and suprasellar space, arising in the posterior pituitary gland. They appear to originate from pituicytes, the resident glial cells of the neurohypophysis (posterior pituitary). Although they are considered to be low-grade neoplasms, their growth causes hormonal and visual disturbances by compressing the pituitary stalk, the anterior pituitary, or the optic chiasm. Because the clinical and imaging features are similar to other, more common sellar or suprasellar masses, the diagnosis of pituicytoma is rarely suspected prior to surgery. Observations made at the time of surgery, on frozen section, or on permanent histology provide clues to the diagnosis. In this chapter, we discuss numerous aspects of pituicytoma, ranging from its apparent pathogenesis to its clinical presentation, diagnosis, and treatment. We also discuss a few emerging areas including molecular genetic features and possible future treatment approaches.

PATHOGENESIS

Pituicytomas are thought to arise from pituicytes of the neurohypophysis. The neurohypophysis contains neuronal axons that descend into the pituitary from the hypothalamus. Pituicytes make up the majority of nucleated cells in this region and are thought to descend from glial lineages [1, 2]. These cells interact with neuronal secretory axons and appear to regulate the release of signaling peptides [2]. Ultrastructural study shows that there are several morphological subtypes of pituicytes, including astrocyte-like, ependymal-like, oncocytic, and granular [1]. No studies have yet revealed molecular distinction or subtype-specific activity.

Many neurons and glial lineages of the ventral forebrain develop from common progenitor cells expressing Thyroid Transcription Factor-1 (TTF-1), encoded by the gene NKX2-1 [3]. Pituicytes retain TTF-1 staining in the adult pituitary [4]. Pituicytomas were also shown to express nuclear TTF-1, supporting the notion that they arise from pituicytes or from a common progenitor [4]. As will be discussed further below, a number of small studies have investigated molecular alterations in pituicytomas and related neoplasms. These entities revealed a variety of genetic and cytogenetic abnormalities [5-7]. When taken together, the molecular data could indicate that pituicytomas result from genetic aberrations in pituicytes or pituicyte progenitor cells. However, a direct lineage relationship has yet to be proven.

Clinical and Imaging Features

Pituicytomas present similarly to other masses of the sellar and suprasellar spaces. Case series and meta-analyses demonstrate a slight male predominance [8, 9]. They also show that the most frequent presenting symptom is visual disturbance, followed by endocrine abnormalities and headaches [8-10]. The reported endocrinopathies mainly include anterior pituitary hormone deficits; hyperprolactinemia, due to compression of the pituitary stalk, is common [8]. Several cases of diabetes insipidus have also been reported [8]. Interestingly, one older meta-analysis did not reveal many cases of diabetes insipidus and suggested that its presence could virtually exclude pituicytoma [10]. It is possible that new cases emerged in the eight years between these two meta-analyses. Alternately, changes in the World Health Organization (WHO) classification system may have caused certain cases to be reclassified as pituicytomas. Regardless of the reason, the results of the more recent meta-analysis suggest that diabetes insipidus should not be used to rule out the presence of a pituicytoma [8].

These two large meta-analyses found similar characteristics of pituicytomas on imaging. One noted that the masses ranged in size from 4-70 millimeters with an average of about 20 mm [8]. On magnetic resonance imaging (MRI), the majority (around 75-80%) showed homogeneous contrast enhancement. The remaining pituicytomas showed heterogeneous enhancement. Most pituicytomas appeared as either suprasellar or mixed sellar/suprasellar masses [8, 10]. Interestingly, a small fraction of pituicytomas were located only in the sellar space. This finding contrasted with other types of posterior pituitary tumors, for which no cases were purely sellar [10]. Isolated sellar location may therefore represent a clue in the differential diagnosis.

HISTOPATHOLOGY

Histologically, pituicytomas consist of sheets of homogeneous spindle cells. The cells are typically bipolar, with long, thin processes extending from either end. They may be arranged either in fascicles or in a radial storiform pattern (Figure 1). There is typically an extensive capillary network within the tumor. This feature correlates with the tendency of these tumors to bleed significantly during surgical removal. Cytologically, the cells of pituicytoma appear bland. There is minimal nuclear atypia, usually including only mild irregularity of the nuclear borders (Figure 2). Mitoses are rare [11]. However, there have been reports of pituicytomas demonstrating nuclear pleomorphism as well as some with more frequent mitoses [4, 7, 12-14]. While these tumors may adhere to adjacent structures, they typically do not infiltrate [11]. Of note, there have also been case reports of pituicytomas showing extensive epithelioid morphology [15, 16].

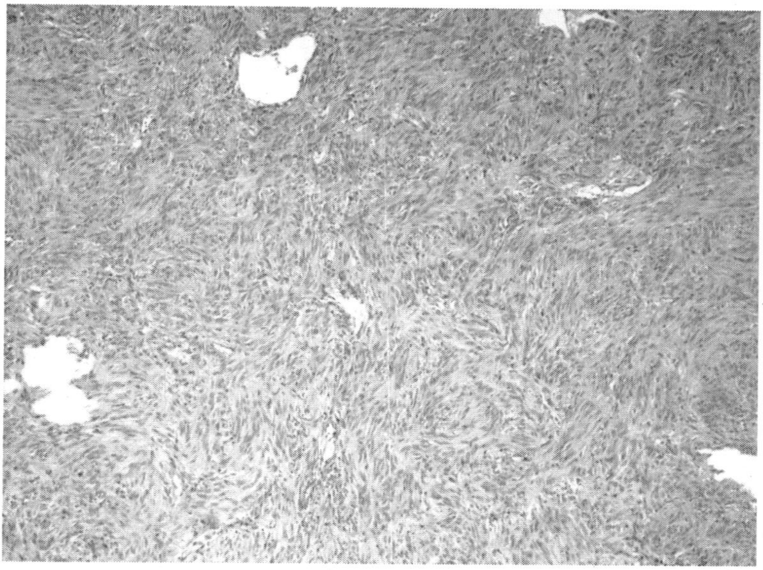

Figure 1. Low magnification appearance of a pituicytoma. The tumor is marked by generally spindled cells arranged in a storiform or fascicular architectural pattern (hematoxylin and eosin, original magnification 100X).

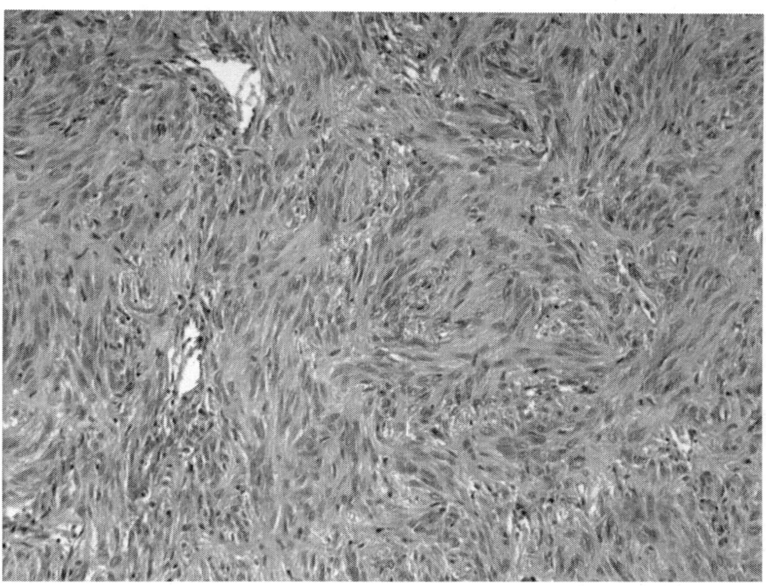

Figure 2. Higher magnification appearance of a pituicytoma. Tumor cells are elongated with mildly irregular nuclear borders and an absence of nucleolation (hematoxylin and eosin, original magnification 200X).

IMMUNOPHENOTYPE

Almost all cases of pituicytoma stain positive for S-100 and vimentin (Figure 3) [11, 15, 17]. These tumors frequently, but not always, exhibit glial fibrillary acidic protein (GFAP) staining. When present, GFAP tends to stain weakly and heterogeneously (Figure 4) [11, 15, 17]. A smaller fraction of pituicytomas stain for epithelial membrane antigen (EMA); when they do, the antigen is primarily detected in the cytoplasm (Figure 5) [11, 15, 17]. As noted previously, pituicytomas have also been shown to display strong nuclear TTF-1 staining (Figure 6) [4, 18]. Pituicytomas do not express neuroendocrine markers such as synaptophysin or neurofilament, a feature that is important for differential diagnostic purposes. Tumors typically demonstrate low labeling indices with cell proliferation markers Ki-67 or MIB-1 (Figure 7).

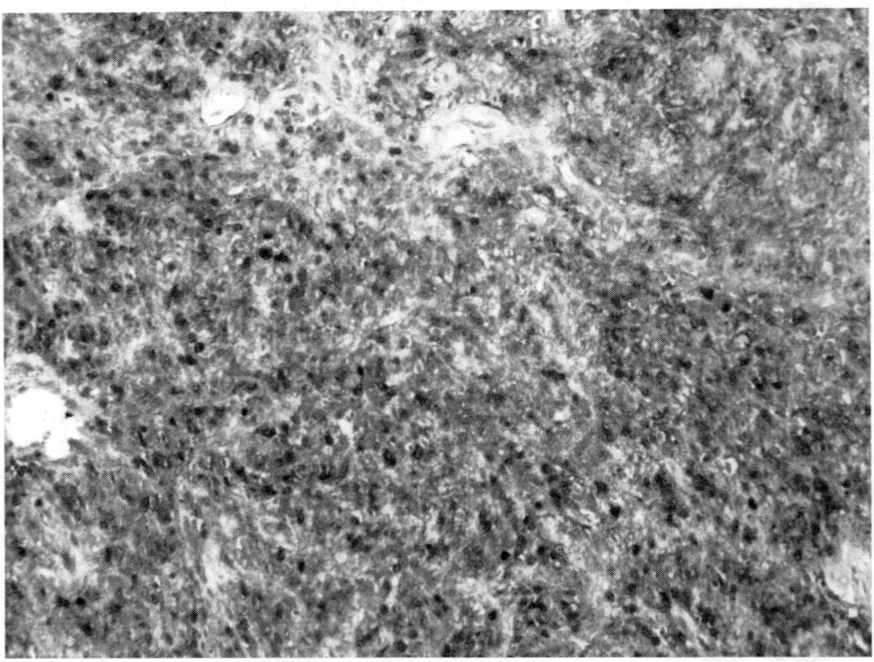

Figure 3. Pituicytomas generally demonstrate diffuse strong immunoreactivity with antibody to S-100 protein (original magnification 200X).

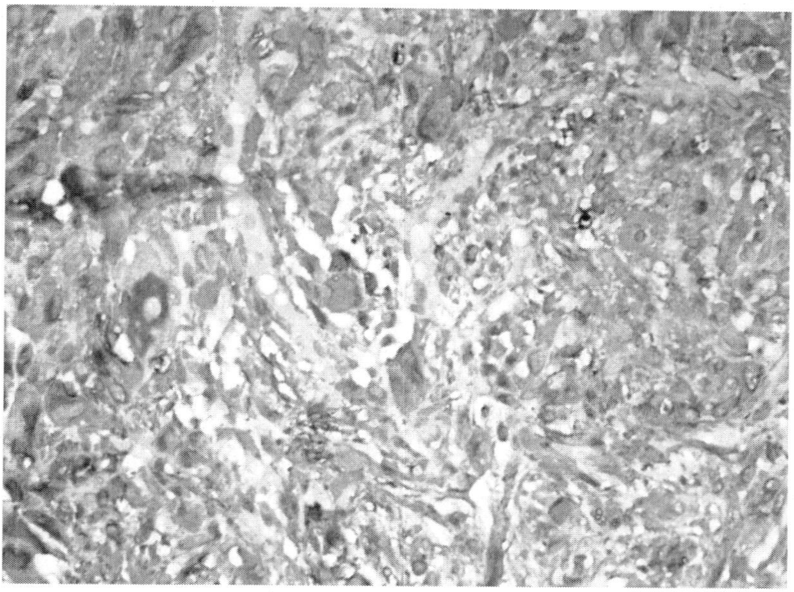

Figure 4. Patchy glial fibrillary acidic protein (GFAP) immunoreactivity may be seen in some pituicytomas (original magnification 400X).

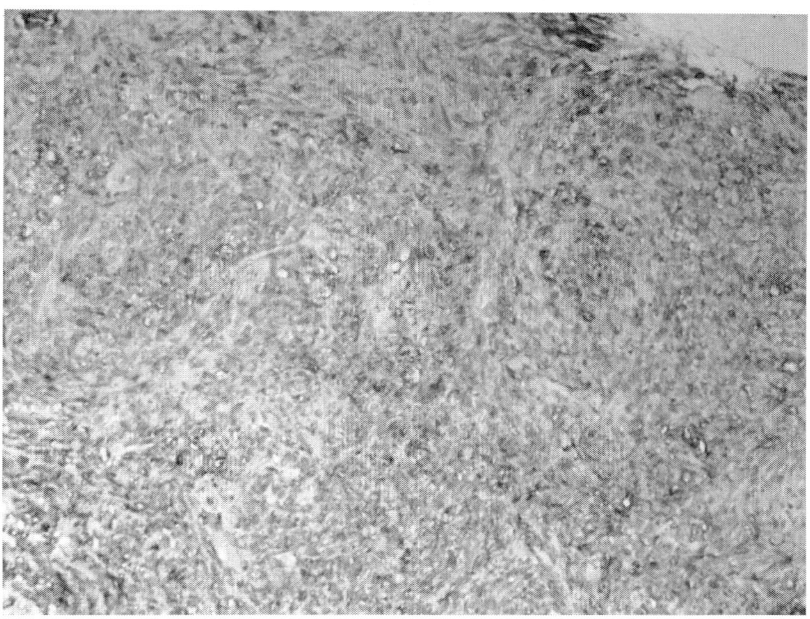

Figure 5. Patchy cytoplasmic epithelial membrane antigen (EMA) immunostaining may be encountered in a subset of pituicytomas (original magnification 200X).

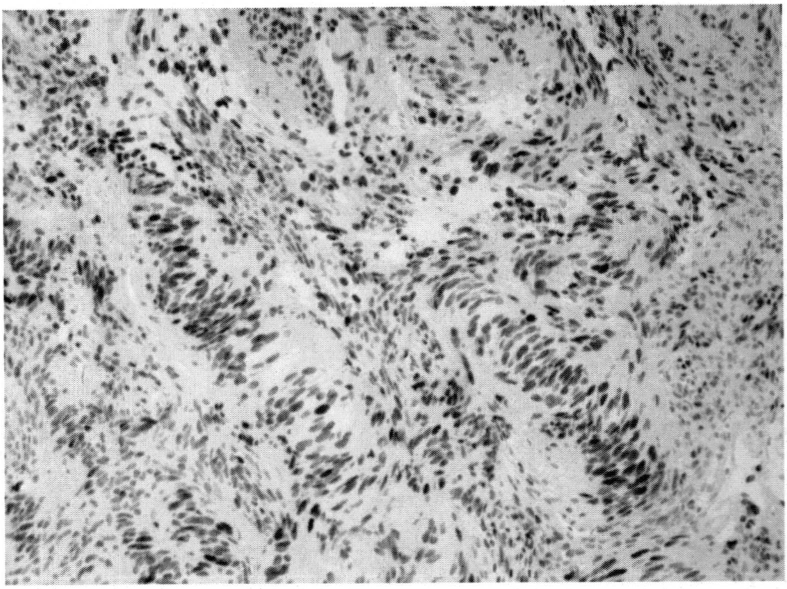

Figure 6. Pituicytoma showing diffuse strong nuclear staining with antibody to thyroid transcription factor-1 (TTF-1) (original magnification 200X).

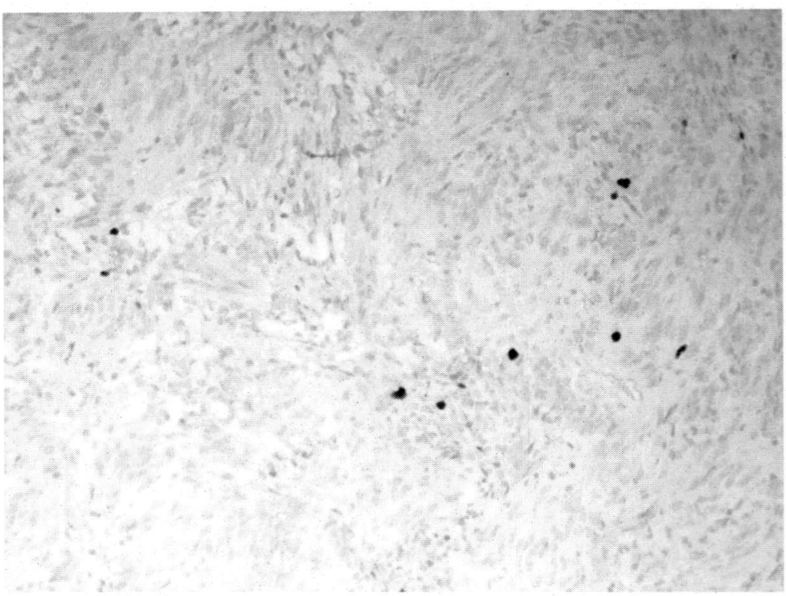

Figure 7. Pituicytomas typically have a low Ki-67 labeling index. Occasional positive staining tumor cells staining with Ki-67 are seen here (original magnification 200X).

Molecular Features

To date, no comprehensive characterization of pituicytoma genetics has been reported. However, a few groups have performed limited molecular studies. One group used array-based genomic hybridization to examine chromosomal abnormalities in one pituicytoma. They found a number of cytogenetic abnormalities, including losses on chromosomes 1p, 14q, and 22q, as well as gains on chromosome 5p [5]. Another group performed immunohistochemical staining for mutations known to be associated with other glial neoplasms; none of the specimens stained positively for IDH1-R132H, BRAF-V600E, or for BRAF-KIAA fusion protein [18]. Most recently, a third group reported results of next-generation sequencing for three cases of pituicytoma. Among a number of findings, the authors reported disease-associated variants in *HRAS* in one tumor, and *BRAF* (V600E), *NF1*, and *TSC1* in another [7]. Immunostaining confirmed the presence of mutant BRAF-V600E. Noting a number of alterations in the MAPK pathway, the authors stained all cases in their series for pERK. All but one case showed strong positive pERK staining, in contrast to weak or absent staining in normal pituitary tissue [7]. Of note, a similar recent study examined spindle cell oncocytomas, a neoplasm related to pituicytoma. The authors reported MAPK pathway alterations and strong pERK staining among several specimens [6]. Taken together, these results suggest MAPK pathway alterations may be highly common among pituicytomas and related neoplasms. Although a pathogenic role for this pathway might be suggested, further work will be required to support such a claim.

Differential Diagnosis

The differential diagnosis for pituicytoma is typically straightforward. Perhaps the greatest challenge is considering it at all when examining sellar neoplasms, since other entities are far more common. For this reason, we will briefly consider several of the more common entities, even though they do not usually resemble pituicytomas histologically. The presence of a homogeneous spindle cell population should trigger suspicion for pituicytoma or its related neoplasms. Once suspected, the characteristic immunohistochemical profile can help reach the correct diagnosis.

Adenoma

Adenomas of the anterior pituitary are far more common than pituicytomas. Typical adenomas appear as sheets of monotonous plump cells, lacking the organized acinar pattern of normal adenohypophyseal tissue. A variety of morphologic variants have been described. Synaptophysin staining should be uniformly and strongly positive, while TTF-1 should be uniformly negative. Many adenomas also stain for one or more anterior pituitary hormones. Lack of this normal staining pattern should raise suspicion for an alternate tumor type [19].

Pilocytic Astrocytoma

Although sellar pilocytic astrocytomas are not especially common, there was once significant confusion between these tumors and pituicytomas, mainly due to inconsistencies with nomenclature [11]. The elongated fibrillar cells of a pilocytic astrocytoma do bear some resemblance to the spindled cells of pituicytoma. However, other characteristic features of pilocytic astrocytomas, such as Rosenthal fibers and eosinophilic granular bodies, are absent in pituicytoma. Herring bodies, normal axonal structures that appear in the posterior pituitary and may therefore be associated with pituicytoma, must not be misinterpreted for eosinophilic granular bodies [19]. Pilocytic astrocytomas should demonstrate diffuse positive GFAP staining, in contrast to the weak, patchy, or absent staining in pituicytoma. Conversely, pilocytic astrocytomas should not stain with TTF-1.

Meningioma

There are numerous morphologic variants of meningioma. The most common variant, the syncytial or meningotheliomatous meningioma, displays rounded cells with abundant cytoplasm and indistinct borders arranged in small clumps. This entity is unlikely to be mistaken or confused with a possible pituicytoma. However, the fibrous/fibroblastic or transitional/mixed meningioma variants do have prominent spindle cell components. Special stains may be required to differentiate these meningioma variants from posterior pituitary lesions. Meningiomas should be strongly and diffusely positive for EMA in a membranous pattern, in contrast with the weaker, patchier, and cytoplasmic staining in pituicytoma. Meningiomas may also be positive for progesterone receptor and SSTR2a. Furthermore, meningiomas should not be TTF-1 positive [19].

Schwannoma

Although schwannomas are unusual tumors to arise in the sella, their spindled cells may resemble those of pituicytomas. Schwannomas classically have distinct regional variation, with recognizable Antoni A and Antoni B areas and occasional palisaded nuclei (Verocay bodies). Pituicytomas are typically more homogeneous. If special stains are ordered to help differentiate these two diagnoses, one must take care, because both will stain strongly for S-100. Schwannomas, however, should be negative for TTF-1 [19].

Metastatic Tumors

Metastases to the pituitary gland are rare [19, 20]. However, were a patient to have a pituitary mass and a synchronous or asynchronous TTF-1 positive carcinoma of the lung or thyroid, it could represent a diagnostic dilemma. Such tumors may be readily distinguishable from pituicytoma based on morphology alone. However, additional stains such as thyroglobulin, Napsin A, or S-100 may be helpful in narrowing or confirming the diagnosis.

Other TTF-1 Positive Lesions

Finally, pituicytomas may be distinguished from other TTF-1 positive spindle cell tumors of the posterior pituitary gland. Pituitary granular cell tumors and spindle cell oncocytomas also display TTF-1 staining and have an overall spindle cell-like morphology [17, 21, 22]. As the names imply, these tumors have unique morphologic characteristics. Pituitary granular cell tumors are similar to those found elsewhere in the body, exhibiting abundant cytoplasm containing numerous discrete eosinophilic granules. Ultrastructural examination confirms that these granules represent lysosomes. Spindle cell oncocytomas have a slightly larger cytoplasm than pituicytomas. The cytoplasm is finely granular, reflecting an increased number of mitochondria. Of note, it has been suggested that these three entities are in fact all variants of pituicytoma [18]. As noted above, ultrastructural examination of the normal neurohypophysis reveals several subtypes of pituicytes, including granular and oncocytic varieties [1]. It has therefore been suggested that each of these posterior pituitary tumors arises from (or mimics) a distinct type of pituicyte [18]. For the time being, WHO classification systems for both central nervous system and endocrine tumors maintain these three tumor types as separate entities [17, 23-26].

Morphology should be sufficient to differentiate these three tumor types in most cases. If immunostains are required, TTF-1 and S-100 will not be helpful, since all three of these entities stain positively. Most cases of pituitary granular cell tumors will stain positively for PAS, unlike pituicytomas or spindle cell oncocytomas. Most spindle cell oncocytomas stain positively for EMA, in a much stronger fashion than pituicytomas [17, 18]. A combination of these markers may therefore help navigate the differential diagnosis in difficult cases.

TREATMENT

Pituicytomas are considered to be grade I lesions by both the central nervous system (CNS) and endocrine WHO criteria [23-28]. Their main threat to the patient derives from local effects of tumors compressing adjacent structures. Notably, some cases of pituicytoma have displayed spontaneous hemorrhage [29]. The main goals of treatment are to alleviate symptoms, prevent progressive deficits, and to avoid complications.

Virtually all reported cases of pituicytoma have been treated surgically. Both trans-sphenoidal and transcranial approaches have been described [8]. Surgeons commonly report extensive bleeding from the lesions during resection. As noted previously, bleeding correlates with the extensive tumor vascularity. Because sellar tumors are usually suspected to be adenomas preoperatively, bleeding may be the first sign that a tumor is in fact a pituicytoma. In some cases, bleeding limits the extent to which tumors can be safely resected. A few groups have performed preoperative embolization to reduce bleeding risk [7, 8]. Relatively high postoperative morbidity rates have been reported. However, the morbidities are mostly mild, persistent endocrinopathies that can be treated [7-9].

Reported cases and case series have had differing degrees and lengths of follow-up. However, the available evidence shows that pituicytoma recurrence is not uncommon. In most cases, recurrence correlates with the degree of resection. Most recurrences occur when the tumors cannot be entirely grossly excised. Notably, the converse is not as reliably true - although many subtotally resected tumors recur, by no means do all recur [8, 9, 30]. When total resection is not possible, radiation therapy may be used to control growth of the residual tumor. In some cases, residual or recurrent tumors remain stable for long periods of time. Unfortunately, a number of patients have experienced devastating complications from reoperations or salvage radiation procedures for recurrent pituicytomas [7, 31].

Systemic therapies have not been extensively described for pituicytoma. At least one case of residual tumor has been treated with chemotherapy. That patient achieved stable disease [4]. At least one study investigated potential targeted therapies. All tumors in the small case series showed strong vascular endothelial growth factor (VEGFR) expression, and most expressed one or more isoforms of the somatostatin receptor (SSTR). Inhibitors of these receptors or downstream signaling pathways may eventually emerge as options for treating pituicytomas and related neoplasms [31]. Unless improved preoperative diagnostic modalities are also developed, it is likely that surgery will remain the standard treatment. However, systemic agents would be especially useful in residual, recurrent, or other problematic cases.

CONCLUSION

The relative rarity of pituicytomas means the index of suspicion must be high in order to arrive at the diagnosis. Through our discussion of pituicytomas, we have highlighted features that provide important diagnostic clues. These include findings on imaging or during resection that, while not specific, may be helpful in raising suspicion. Although histologic features of pituicytomas are not shared by most other sellar tumors, immunohistochemical confirmation is helpful. A limited selection of antibodies that most laboratories carry can reliably narrow the differential diagnosis. Treatment currently consists of surgical resection, which provides satisfactory disease control in most cases. However, when complete resection cannot be achieved, pituicytomas often recur. Emerging molecular understanding may provide additional therapeutic avenues in the future.

REFERENCES

[1] Takei, Y., Seyama, S., Pearl, G.S., and Tindall, G.T. (1980). Ultrastructural study of the human neurohypophysis. II. Cellular elements of neural parenchyma, the pituicytes. *Cell Tissue Res.* 205(2): 273-87.

[2] Hatton, G.I. (1988). Pituicytes, glia and control of terminal secretion. *J. Exp. Biol.* 139: 67-79.

[3] Turrero García, M., and Harwell, C.C. (2017). Radial glia in the ventral telencephalon. *FEBS Lett.* 591(24): 3942-59.

[4] Lee, E.B., Tihan, T., Scheithauer, B.W., Zhang, P.J., and Gonatas, N.K. (2009). Thyroid transcription factor 1 expression in sellar tumors: a histogenetic marker? *J. Neuropathol. Exp. Neurol.* 68(5): 482-8.

[5] Phillips, J.J., Misra, A., Feuerstein, B.G., Kunwar, S., and Tihan, T. (2010). Pituicytoma: characterization of a unique neoplasm by histology, immunohistochemistry, ultrastructure, and array-based comparative genomic hybridization. *Arch. Pathol. Lab. Med.* 134(7): 1063-9.

[6] Miller, M.B., Bi, W.L., Ramkissoon, L.A., Kang, Y.J., Abedalthagafi, M., Knoff, D.S., Agarwalla, P.K., et al. (2016). MAPK activation and HRAS mutation identified in pituitary spindle cell oncocytoma. *Oncotarget.* 7(24): 37054-63.

[7] Viaene, A.N., Lee, E.B., Rosenbaum, J.N., Nasrallah, I.M., and Nasrallah, M.P. (2019). Histologic, immunohistochemical, and molecular features of pituicytomas and atypical pituicytomas. *Acta Neuropathol. Commun.* 7(1): 69.

[8] Salge-Arrieta, F.J., Carrasco-Moro, R., Rodríguez-Berrocal, V., Pian, H., Martínez-San Millán, J.S., Iglesias, P., and Ley-Urzáiz, L. (2019). Clinical features, diagnosis and therapy of pituicytoma: an update. *J. Endocrinol. Invest.* 42(4): 371-384.

[9] Pirayesh Islamian, A., Buslei, R., Saeger, W., and Fahlbusch, R. (2012). Pituicytoma: overview of treatment strategies and outcome. *Pituitary.* 15(2): 227-36.

[10] Covington, M.F., Chin, S.S., and Osborn, A.G. (2011). Pituicytoma, spindle cell oncocytoma, and granular cell tumor: clarification and meta-analysis of the world literature since 1893. *AJNR Am. J. Neuroradiol*. 32(11): 2067-72.

[11] Brat, D.J., Scheithauer, B.W., Staugaitis, S.M., Holtzman, R.N., Morgello, S., and Burger, P.C. (2000). Pituicytoma: a distinctive low-grade glioma of the neurohypophysis. *Am. J. Surg. Pathol*. 24(3): 362-8.

[12] Takei, H., Goodman, J.C., Tanaka, S., Bhattacharjee, M.B., Bahrami, A., and Powell, S.Z. (2005). Pituicytoma incidentally found at autopsy. *Pathol. Int*. 55(11): 745-9.

[13] Kwon, M.J. and Suh, Y.L. (2011). Pituicytoma with unusual histological features. *Pathol. Int*. 61(10): 598-602.

[14] Zhi, L., Yang, L., Quan, H., and Bai-ning, L. (2009). Pituicytoma presenting with atypical histological features. *Pathology*. 41(5): 505-9.

[15] Ellis, J.A., Tsankova, N.M., D'Amico, R., Ausiello, J.C., Canoll, P., Rosenblum, M.K., and Bruce, J.N. (2012). Epithelioid pituicytoma. *World Neurosurg*. 78(1-2): 191.E1-7.

[16] Vellutini, E.A.S., Becker, P.H.P., Godoy, L.F., Guerreiro, N.F.C., Mattedi, R.L., and de Oliveira, M.F. (2018). Epithelioid pituicytoma: An unusual case report. *Surg. Neurol. Int*. 9: 145.

[17] Shibuya, M. (2018). Welcoming the new WHO classification of pituitary tumors 2017: revolution in TTF-1-positive posterior pituitary tumors. *Brain Tumor Pathol*. 35(2): 62-70.

[18] Mete, O., Lopes, M.B., and Asa, S.L. (2013). Spindle cell oncocytomas and granular cell tumors of the pituitary are variants of pituicytoma. *Am. J. Surg. Pathol*. 37(11): 1694-9.

[19] Kleinschmidt-DeMasters, B.K., Lopes, M.B., and Prayson, R.A. (2015). An algorithmic approach to sellar region masses. *Arch. Pathol. Lab. Med*. 139(3): 356-72.

[20] He, W., Chen, F., Dalm, B., Kirby, P.A., and Greenlee, J.D. (2015). Metastatic involvement of the pituitary gland: a systematic review with pooled individual patient data analysis. *Pituitary*. 18(1): 159-68.

[21] El Hussein, S. and Vincentelli, C. (2017). Pituicytoma: Review of commonalities and distinguishing features among TTF-1 positive tumors of the central nervous system. *Ann. Diagn. Pathol.* 29: 57-61.

[22] Kleinschmidt-DeMasters, B.K., and Lopes, M.B. (2013). Update on hypophysitis and TTF-1 expressing sellar region masses. *Brain Pathol.* 23(5): 495-514.

[23] Louis, D.N., Perry, A., Reifenberger, G., von Deimling, A., Figarella-Branger, D., Cavenee, W.K., Ohgaki, H., Wiestler, O.D., Kleihues, P., and Ellison, D.W. (2016). The 2016 World Health Organization Classification of Tumors of the Central Nervous System: a summary. *Acta Neuropathol.* 131(6): 803-20.

[24] Mete, O., and Lopes, M.B. (2017). Overview of the 2017 WHO Classification of Pituitary Tumors. *Endocr. Pathol.* 28(3): 228-243.

[25] Lopes, M.B.S. (2017). The 2017 World Health Organization classification of tumors of the pituitary gland: a summary. *Acta Neuropathol.* 134(4): 521-535.

[26] Sahm, F., Reuss, D.E., and Giannini, C. (2018). WHO 2016 classification: changes and advancements in the diagnosis of miscellaneous primary CNS tumours. *Neuropathol. Appl. Neurobiol.* 44(2): 163-171.

[27] Brat, D.J., Scheithauer, B.W., Fuller, G.N., and Tihan, T. (2007). Newly codified glial neoplasms of the 2007 WHO Classification of Tumours of the Central Nervous System: angiocentric glioma, pilomyxoid astrocytoma and pituicytoma. *Brain. Pathol.* 17(3): 319-24.

[28] Louis, D.N., Ohgaki, H., Wiestler, O.D., Cavenee, W.K., Burger, P.C., Jouvet, A., Scheithauer, B.W., and Kleihues, P. (2007). The 2007 WHO classification of tumours of the central nervous system. *Acta Neuropathol.* 114(2): 97-109.

[29] Benveniste, R.J., Purohit D., and Byun, H. (2006). Pituicytoma presenting with spontaneous hemorrhage. *Pituitary.* 9(1): 53-8.

[30] Lefevre, E., Bouazza, S., Bielle, F., and Boch, A.L. (2018). Management of pituicytomas: a multicenter series of eight cases. *Pituitary*. 21(5): 507-514.

[31] Mende, K.C., Matschke, J., Burkhardt, T., Saeger, W., Buslei, R., Buchfelder, M., Fahlbusch, R., Westphal, M., and Flitsch, J. (2017) Pituicytoma-An outlook on possible targeted therapies. *CNS Neurosci. Ther*. 23(7): 620-626.

In: The Pituitary Gland and Adrenal Glands ISBN: 978-1-53617-605-6
Editor: Noémi Barta

Chapter 2

SPINDLE CELL ONCOCYTOMAS OF THE PITUITARY GLAND

Diana Basali, MD and Richard A. Prayson*, MD, MEd
Departments of Internal Medicine and Anatomic Pathology*,
Cleveland Clinic, Cleveland, OH, US

ABSTRACT

In 2002, Roncaroli et al. reported the first 5 cases of a mitochondrial-rich, spindled cell tumor presumably arising in the adenohypophysis of the pituitary gland. They coined the name "spindle cell oncocytoma." For the entity. Spindle cell oncocytomas are rare tumors, accounting for less than 0.5% of sellar masses. Tumors typically present in adults and most commonly manifest with visual disturbances and pituitary hypofunction. On imaging and gross inspection, these tumors may resemble pituitary adenomas. Microscopically, they are marked by interlacing fascicles of spindled cells with eosinophilic cytoplasm. Tumors may demonstrate some degree of nuclear atypia. Cell proliferation rates are low. These tumors do not express neuroendocrine and hormonal immunomarkers typically seen in pituitary adenomas. They do express S-100 protein, EMA and BCL2 immunoreactivity. Similar to pituicytomas and granular

* Corresponding Author's E-mail: praysor@ccf.org.

cell tumors, they also show evidence of thyroid transcription factor-1 (TTF-1) immunoreactivity, suggesting that these tumors may in fact originate from pituicytes in the neurohypophysis of the gland. Spindle cell oncocytomas are considered to be benign (World Health Organization grade I neoplasms). A subset of tumors have been reported to recur after several years, particularly if incompletely resected. This chapter will review the clinical and pathologic features of these neoplasms.

INTRODUCTION

Spindle cell oncocytoma of the pituitary was first recognized as a distinct entity in 2002 by Roncaroli and colleagues [1]. They described five adult patients who had tumors which they ascribed to arising in the anterior pituitary gland [1]. The tumors, on neuroimaging, showed evidence of suprasellar extension and looked like pituitary adenomas. They were marked by spindled cells with cytoplasm rich in mitochondria. No recurrences were noted in the gross totally resected tumors. They hypothesized that spindle cell oncocytomas arose from folliculostellate cells located in the adenohypophysis of the pituitary gland.

More recent studies have shown that these tumors demonstrate thyroid transcription factor-1 (TTF-1) immunostaining [2, 3]. Similar staining with TTF-1 has been noted to occur in pituicytes situated in the neurohypophysis or posterior pituitary gland, suggesting that these tumors may arise in that location, rather than the anterior portion of the gland, as initially postulated by Roncaroli et al. [1]. A similar pattern of immunoreactivity has been observed with granular cell tumors and pituicytomas of the pituitary gland, leading some to conjecture that the three tumors may be related lesions [3]. The morphologic variability of these three tumors may reflect the fact that there appears to be multiple subtypes of pituicytes in the normal neurohypophysis [3, 4]. In their ultrastructural study of the posterior pituitary, Takei et al. noted five variants of pituicytes: dark, light, ependymal, oncocytic and granular [4]. This may account for the phenotypic variability observed in the tumors arising from these cells.

Clinical Presentation

In the original Roncaroli et al. study, two of the five reported tumors came from one institution and comprised 0.4% of all the sellar region masses excised over a 10 year period [1]. In a recent report, it has been asserted that there are less than 50 cases of the entity reported in the literature [5-7]. Most tumors have arisen in adults, with a mean age of 56 years and there appears to be no obvious gender predilection [8-10].

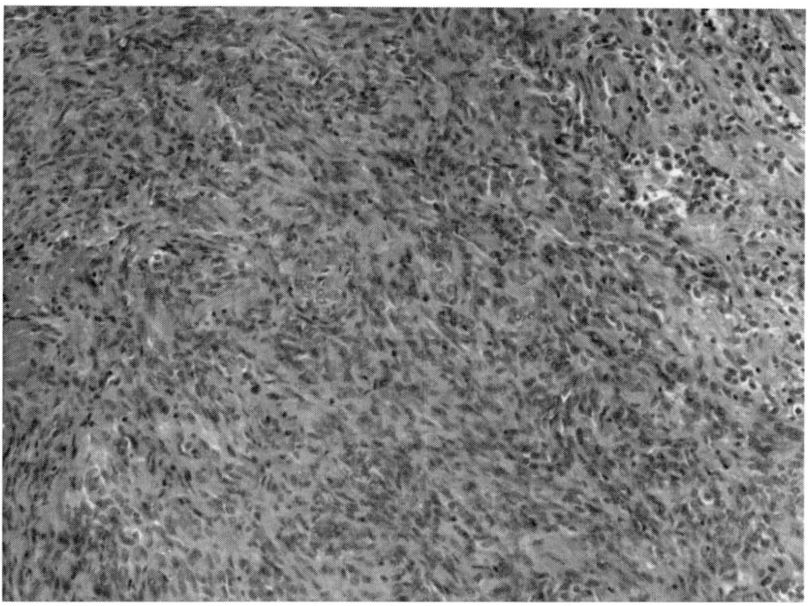

Figure 1. A spindle cell oncocytoma marked by interlacing fascicles of elongated cells with eosinophilic cytoplasm (hematoxylin and eosin, original magnification 200X).

Most tumors arise in the pituitary gland but may occupy space in both the sellar and suprasellar regions. Intrasellar tumors are typically clinically asymptomatic; tumors which extend beyond the sella are more commonly symptomatic [11]. Rarely, tumors may extend to involve the cavernous sines or invade the floor of the sella [12-14]. The most common presenting symptoms are visual disturbances related to mass effect; other less commonly encountered presentations include pituitary dysfunction, nausea, vomiting, and headaches [1, 6, 10, 11, 15]. Rare tumors have unusual presentations including epistaxis and symptoms related to pituitary stalk compression (sexual dysfunction, decreased libido and menstrual abnormalities [9, 14].

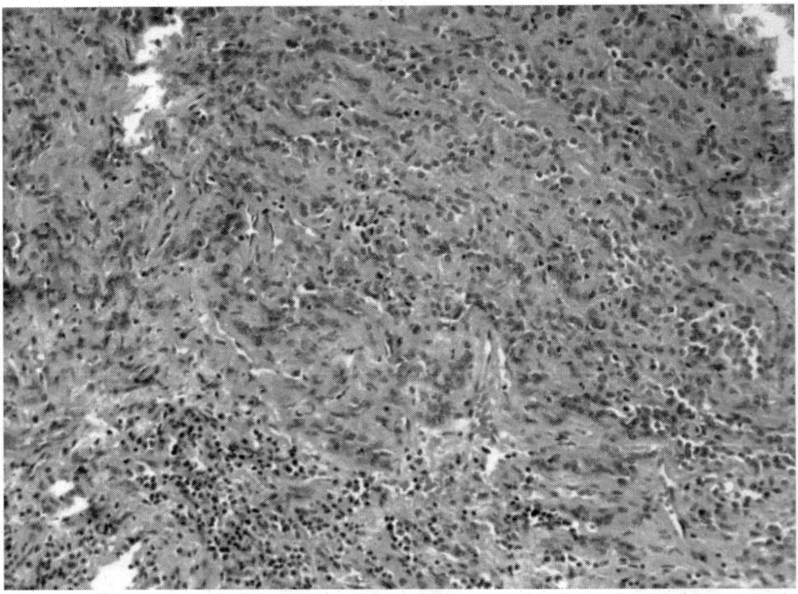

Figure 2. Focal fibrosis and benign perivascular lymphocytes may be encountered in a spindle cell oncocytoma (original magnification 200X).

On imaging, spindle cell oncocytomas look similar to pituitary adenomas but are more likely to show heterogenous enhancement on magnetic resonance imaging (MRI) [8, 11]. Calcifications may occasionally be identified in the tumor on imaging [16]. Intratumoral bleeding in the tumor can create an imaging appearance reminiscent of a craniopharyngioma [16].

Grossly, tumors range from soft to firm and may adhere to surrounding structures, A clear margin of resection, more typically a feature of adenomas, is often not visible.

PATHOLOGY

Microscopically, spindle cell oncocytomas are marked by spindled to epithelioid cells, arranged in interlacing fascicles (Figure 1). Cells are often marked by eosinophilic cytoplasm and may sometimes show oncocytic and/or clear cell changes. Nuclear atypia and pleomorphism may be encountered. Architectural features that may be variably encountered include myxoid change, fibrosis, whorling, osteoclastic giant cells and follicle-like structures [8, 17-19] (Figure 20). Benign appearing perivascular lymphocytes may sometimes be encountered (Figure 2) and some tumors show evidence of calcification (Figure 3). Mitotic activity is minimal in most tumors; occasional recurrent tumors have demonstrated increase mitotic activity [9, 14]. As previously mentioned, intratumoral hemorrhage/hemosiderin [16] may be present. Necrosis has also been rarely described [20].

In contrast to pituitary adenomas, spindle cell oncocytomas do not stain with neuroendocrine markers (synaptophysin, neuron specific enolase, chromogranin) or pituitary hormone markers [8]. Positive staining with a host of immunomarkers has been described including vimentin, S-100 protein, BCL2, epithelial membrane antigen (EMA), MU213-UC clone 131-1 (antimitochondrial antibody), TTF-1, glial fibrillary acidic protein (GFAP), CD44, nestin, galectin-3 and annexin [1-3, 5, 6, 8, 10, 14, 16, 21] (Figures 4 and 5). Cell proliferation markers, such as MIB-1 or Ki-67, show generally low labeling indices in the 1-8% range [8] (Figure 6). Rare cases of recurrent [14, 20] tumors have shown markedly elevated labeling indices, as high as 45%.

Molecular and genetic information about spindle cell oncocytomas is limited. Of the seven tumors evaluated by Mete et al., none of them demonstrated evidence of a BRAF V600E alteration or a BRAF-KIAA fusion [3], similar to what was seen in the pituicytomas and granular cell tumors of the pituitary, which were also studied.

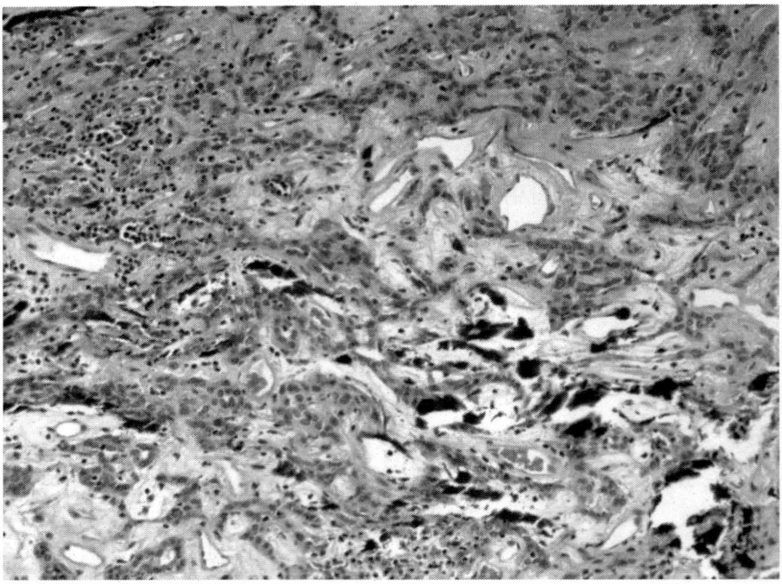

Figure 3. Focal fibrosis and calcification in a spindle cell oncocytoma (hematoxylin and eosin, original magnification 200X).

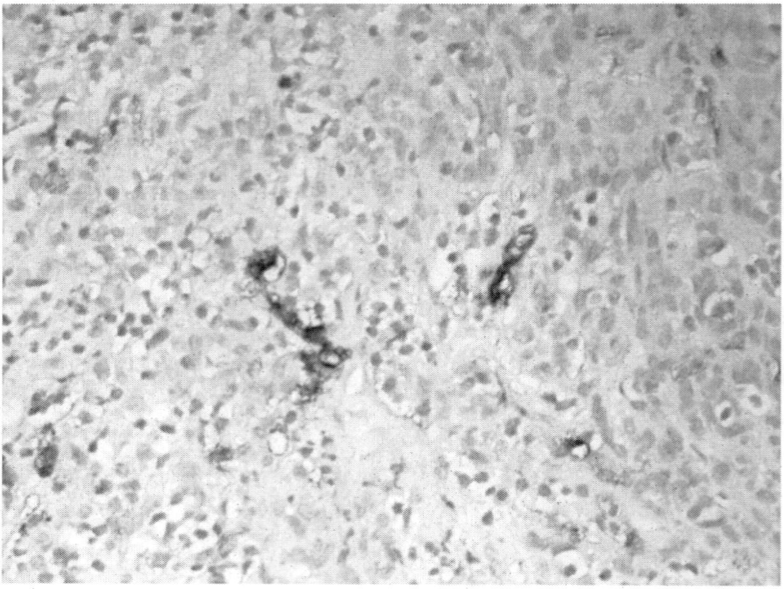

Figure 4. Focal S-100 protein immunoreactivity is commonly seen in these tumors (original magnification 400X).

DIFFERENTIAL DIAGNOSIS

From an imaging perspective and given the prevalence of lesions in the pituitary, the major differential diagnostic consideration is a pituitary adenoma. Adenomas are often (but not always) associated with hormonal production, can present with symptoms related to hormone production and will stain with neuroendocrine markers or with antibodies to the pituitary hormones. TTF-1 immunostaining is not a feature of pituitary adenoma.

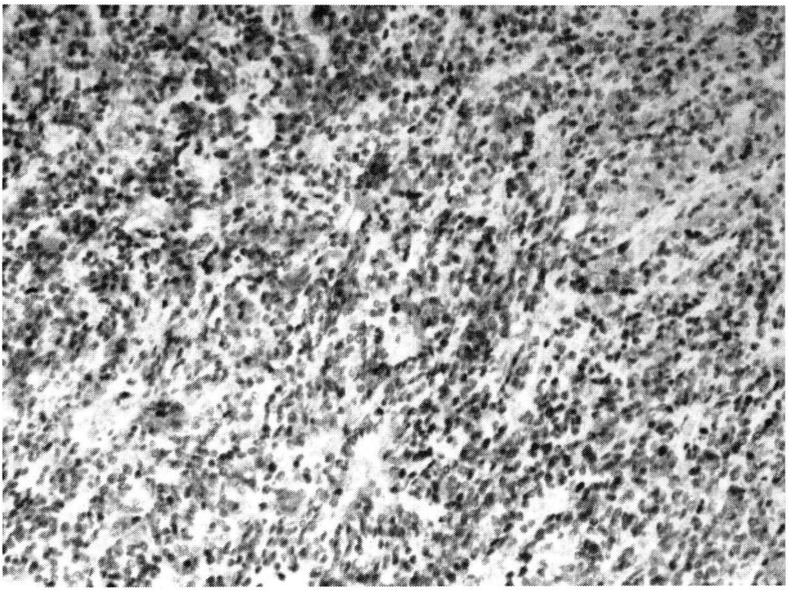

Figure 5. Diffuse nuclear positive staining with antibody to thyroid transcription factor-1 (TTF-1) is a characteristic feature of the tumor (hematoxylin and eosin, original magnification 200X).

Meningiomas arising in the region and present as circumscribed masses and at times can be comprised of cells with an oncocytic-type cytoplasm [22]. Like spindle cell oncocytomas, they may also stain with antibodies to vimentin and EMA and S-100 protein.

In contrast, meningiomas frequently demonstrate immunostaining to progesterone receptor antibody (PR) and somatostatin receptor 2a (SSTR2a) and do not stain with TTF-1 antibody. Low grade solitary fibrous tumor/hemangiopericytoma can also arise rarely in this region [23]. Tumor cells tend to be more spindled with collagen deposition between individual cells. STAT 6 antibody is a reliable marker of solitary fibrous tumor/hemangiopericytoma; TTF-1 immunostaining is not a feature of solitary fibrous tumor/hemangiopericytoma.

Rare cases of schwannomas arising in the sellar region have also been described [24]. Like meningiomas and solitary fibrous tumors/hemangiopericytomas, they also present as a circumscribed mass and are marked by generally spindled cells with compact Antoni A areas juxtaposed with looser Antoni B regions. Nuclear palisading, Verocay bodies, is a feature of some schwannomas and is not seen in spindle cell oncocytomas. Both tumors may stain with S-100 protein. TTF-1 immunoreactivity is not observed in schwannomas.

Although craniopharyngiomas may occasionally resemble, on imaging, spindle cell oncocytoma, the morphology of these tumors is significantly different enough that there is little chance of confusion pathologically, The adamantinomatous craniopharyngioma is marked by nests of epithelioid cells featuring loose or microcytic areas (stellate reticulum), whorling, basal palisading and anucleate pale ghost cells (wet keratin). TTF-1 staining is absent. Papillary craniopharyngiomas are characterized by squamoid type epithelium lining fibrovascular cores.

The two tumors which are most likely to be confused with spindle cell oncocytoma, after pituitary adenoma, are granular cell tumors and pituicytomas. These two neoplasms also arise in the neurohypophysis of the gland from pituicytes and also demonstrate TTF-1 immunoreactivity [3, 11, 25, 26]. Mete and colleagues even went so far as to suggest that spindle cell oncocytomas and granular cell tumors are variants of pituicytoma and they further recommended that spindle cell oncocytoma should be renamed "oncocytic pituicytoma," since they are derived from pituicytes and share TTF-1 immunostaining [3]. The subsequently published WHO guidelines in 2016 has kept the three tumors as separate and distinct entities [8]. Morphologically, granular cell tumors are marked by cells with abundant eosinophilic granular cytoplasm secondary to abundant cytoplasmic lysosomes. Pituicytomas are composed of elongated to rounded cells arranged in fascicles or in a storiform pattern.

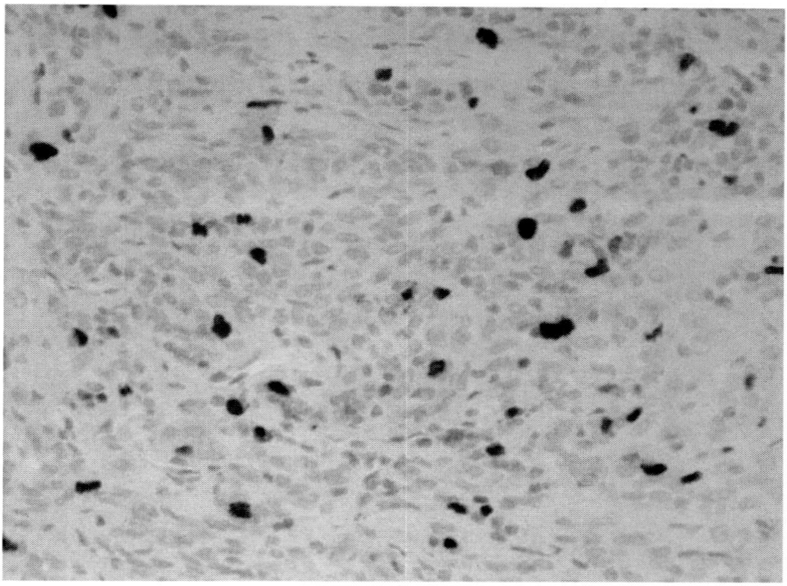

Figure 6. Ki-67 immunostaining typically shows low rates of cell proliferation in these tumors; this particular tumor had a labeling index of 7.5% (original magnification 400x).

Treatment and Prognosis

As suggested by their WHO designation as grade I tumors, the majority of spindle cell oncocytomas have a benign clinical course, although a minority of cases have recurred when subtotally resected [1, 8, 10, 11, 14-16].

As previously indicated, recurrent tumors may have accompanying higher Ki-67 labeling indices. There is no need for adjuvant chemotherapy. Some have reported using radiotherapy in treating some tumors [13, 14, 20]; in some instances, tumor recurrence following radiotherapy was not seen [13] and in other cases, the tumor recurred following radiotherapy [14].

REFERENCES

[1] Roncaroli F, Scheithauer BW, Cenacchi G, Horvath E, Kovacs K, Lloyd RV, Abell-Aleff P, Santi M, Yates AJ. 'Spindle cell oncocytoma' of the adenohypophysis. *Am. J. Surg. Pathol.,* 2002; 26(8): 1048-1055.

[2] Lee EB, Tihan T, Scheithauer BW, Zhang PJ, Gonatas NK. Thyroid transcription factor 1 expression in sellar tumors: a histogenetic marker? *J. Neuropathol. Exp. Neurol.,* 2009; 68(5): 482-488.

[3] Mete O, Lopes MB, Asa SL. Spindle cell oncocytomas and granular cell tumors of the pituitary are variants of pituicytoma. *Am. J. Surg. Pathol.,* 2013; 37(11): 1694-1699.

[4] Takei Y, Seyama S, Pearl GS, Tindall GT. Ultrastructural study of the human neurohypophysis. II. Cellular elements of neural parenchyma, the pituicytes. *Cell Tissue Res.,* 1980; 205(2): 273-287.

[5] Yip CM, Lee HP, Hseih PP. Pituitary spindle cell oncocytoma presented as pituitary apoplexy. *J. Surg. Case Rep.,* 2019; 6: 1-4.

[6] Larsen AMG, Cote DJ, Zaidi HA, Bi WL, Schmitt PJ. Jorgulescu JB, Miller MB, Smith TR, Lopes MB, Jane JA Jr, Laws ER Jr. Spindle cell oncocytoma of the pituitary gland. *J. Neurosurg.,* 2018; DOI: 10.3171/2018.4.JNS18211.

[7] Gupta RK, Batra VV, Singh D, Sharma MC, Kumar V. Is spindle cell oncocytoma a true entity or a variant of pituicytoma? A case report with review of literature. *Neurol. India,* 2018; 66: 1413-1418.

[8] Lopes MBS, Fuller GN, Roncaroli F, Wesseling P. Spindle cell oncocytoma. In: *WHO Classification of Tumours of the Central Nervous System.* Louis DN, Ohgaki H, Wiestler OD, Cavenee WK, Ellison DW, Figarella-Branger D, Perry A, Reifenberger G, von Deimling A. IARC. Lyon, FR. 2016: 334-336.

[9] Mu Q, Yu J, Qu L, Hu X, Gao H, Liu P, Zheng X, Sun Y, Huang H. Spindle cell oncocytoma of the adenohypophysis: two case reports and a review of the literature. *Mol. Med. Rep.,* 2015; 12(1): 871-876.

[10] Sali A, Tampi C, Goel A. Spindle cell oncocytoma of adenohypophysis: Review of literature and report of another recurrent case. *Neuropathology,* 2017; 37: 535-543.

[11] Covington MF, Chin SS, Osborn AG. Pituicytoma, spindle cell oncocytoma, and granular cell tumor: Clarification and meta-analysis of the world literature since 1893. *Am. J. Neuroradiol.,* 2011; 32: 2067-2072.

[12] Borota OC, Scheithauer BW, Fougner SL, Hald JK, Ramm-Pettersen J, Bollerslev J. Spindle cell oncocytoma of the adenohypophysis: report of a case with marked cellular atypia and recurrence despite adjuvant treatment. *Clin. Neuropathol.,* 2009; 28(2): 91-95.

[13] Dahiya S, Sarkar C, Hedley-Whyte ET, Sharma MC, Zervas NT, Sridhar E, Louis DN. Spindle cell oncocytoma of the adenohypophysis: report of two cases. *Acta Neuropathol.,* 2005; 110(1): 97-99.

[14] Kloub O, Perry A, Tu PH, Lipper M, Lopes MB. Spindle cell oncocytoma of the adenohypophysis: report of two recurrent cases. *Am. J. Surg. Pathol.,* 2005; 29(2): 247-253.

[15] Demissie YN, Joseph J, Dawson T, Roberts G, de Carpentier J, Howell S. Recurrent spindle cell oncocytoma of the pituitary, a case report and review of the literature. *Pituitary,* 2011; 14: 367-370.

[16] Borges MT, Lillehei KO, Kleinschmidt-DeMasters BK. Spindle cell oncocytoma with late recurrence and unique neuroimaging characteristics due to recurrent subclinical intratumoral bleeding. *J. Neurooncol.,* 2011; 101(1): 145-154.

[17] Rotman JA, Kucharczyk W, Zadeh G, Kiehl TR, Al-Ahmadi H. Spindle cell oncocytoma of the adenohypophysis: a case report illustrating its natural history with 8-year observation and a review of the literature. *Clin. Imaging,* 2014; 38(4): 499-504.

[18] Vajtai I, Beck J, Kappeler A, Hewer E. Spindle cell oncocytoma of the pituitary gland with follicle-like component: organotypic differentiation to support its origin from folliculo-stellate cells. *Acta Neuropathol.,* 2011; 122(2): 253-258.

[19] Yoshimoto T, Takahashi-Fujigasaki J, Inoshita N, Fukuhara N, Nishioka H, Yamada S. TTF-1 positive oncocytic sellar tumor with follicle formation/ependymal differentiation: non-adenomatous tumor capable of two different interpretations as a pituicytoma or a spindle cell oncocytoma. *Brain Tumor Pathol.*, 2015; 32(3): 221-227.

[20] Kong X, Li D, Kong Y, Zhong D. Malignant adenohypophysis spindle cell oncocytoma with repeating recurrences and a high Ki-67 index. *Medicine,* 2017; 96: 4(e5657).

[21] Romero-Rojas AE, Melo-Uribe MA, Barajas-Solano PA, Chinchilla-Olaya SI, Escobar LI, Hernandez-Walteros DM. Spindle cell oncocytoma of the adenohypophysis. *Brain Tumor Pathol.*, 2011; 28(4): 359-364.

[22] Kwancharoen R, Blitz AM, Tavares F, Caturegli P, Gallia GL, Salvatori R. Clinical features of sellar and suprasellar meningiomas. *Pituitary,* 2014; 17(4): 342-348.

[23] Yang X, Jiang Q, Yu B. Solitary fibrous tumor located in the sella turcica: A report of two cases and review of the literature. *Oncol. Letters,* 2015; 10: 354-358.

[24] Mohammed S, Kovacs K, Munoz D, Cusimano A. A short illustrated review of sellar region schwannoma. *Acta Neurochir. (Wein),* 2010; 152: 885-891.

[25] Brat DJ, Scheithauer BW, Staugaitis SM, Holtzman RN, Morgello S, Burger PC. Pituicytomas: a distinctive low-grade glioma of the neurohypophysis. *Am. J. Surg. Pathol.,* 2000; 24(3): 362-368.

[26] Cohen-Gadol AA, Pichelmann MA, Link MJ, Scheithauer BW, Krecke KN, Young WF Jr, Giannini C. Granular cell tumor of the sellar and suprasellar region: clinicopathologic study of 11 cases and literature review. *Mayo Clin. Proc.,* 2003; 78(5): 567-573.

In: The Pituitary Gland and Adrenal Glands ISBN: 978-1-53617-605-6
Editor: Noémi Barta

Chapter 3

Mixed Gangliocytoma-Pituitary Adenoma of the Pituitary Gland

Richard A. Prayson*[*]*, MD, MEd
Cleveland Clinic Department of Anatomic Pathology,
Cleveland, OH, US

Abstract

Gangliocytomas are rare benign tumors of the neuroaxis. They most commonly arise in children and young adults and most often arise in the cerebellum as part of Cowden's disease (Lhermitte-Duclos disease) or in the sellar region. Isolated sellar gangliocytomas comprise about 0.3-0.5% of all sellar lesions. A subset of sellar gangliocytomas have been described in association with pituitary adenomas; these mixed tumors comprise about 0.5-1.25% of all sellar region tumors. Most of these combined tumors are associated with endocrinopathies, most commonly acromegaly. Multiple theories have been proposed regarding the histogenesis of these mixed tumors. This chapter will review the clinical and pathologic features of these rare mixed tumors and discuss the proposed theories behind their origin.

[*] Corresponding Author's E-mail: praysor@ccf.org.

INTRODUCTION

Gangliocytomas are rare, generally low grade tumors, marked by irregular clusters of neuronal or ganglionic cells, often showing dysplastic features [1]. These tumors are designated by the World Health Organization (WHO) as grade I neoplasms [1]. In isolation, they most frequently are diagnosed in children in associated with pharmacoresistent epilepsy [2] or are encountered in the cerebellum where they are referred to as dysplastic cerebellar gangliocytomas (Lhermitte-Duclos disease); Lhermitte Duclos disease is associated with PTEN mutations and Cowden syndrome [3, 4]. The Lhermitte-Duclos lesion is felt by some to represent a hamartomatous lesion rather than a true neoplasm [5]. The focus of this chapter is on gangliocytomas that arise in the region of the sella in association with pituitary adenomas. Gangliocytomas arising in the posterior pituitary gland are rare. They may arise as isolated tumors but the majority are part of composite lesions, so-called mixed gangliocytoma-pituitary adenoma. The term "pituitary adenoma with adenohypophyseal neuronal choristoma" has also been used by some in the past for this mixed neoplasm [6].

CLINICAL PRESENTATION

Pure gangliocytomas originating in the sellar region account for less than 1% of sellar tumors [7]. In a study of 4122 of pituitary tumors, only 14 (0.34%) tumors were gangliocytomas; 13 out of 14 of the cases were associated with an adenoma [7]. Gangliocytomas have been associated with pituitary adenomas in about two-thirds of cases in the sellar region in other series [8-10]. Pure pituitary adenomas are the most common tumor to arise in the sellar region, where they comprise about 10-15% of all primary brain tumors [11].

Most of the combined tumors present with signs and symptoms related to production of pituitary hormones. Most commonly, the adenomatous component in this setting is associated with production of growth hormone and acromegaly/gigantism [6, 9, 12-15]. Less commonly, patients, may present with an adenomatous component that produces other hormones and signs and symptoms accordingly, including hypercortisolism and hyperprolactinemia [13-20]. Mixed tumors may occasionally present with other signs and symptoms, most commonly including visual disturbances, headaches, or dysmenorrhea [13].

In an analysis of 95 cases of mixed gangliocytoma-pituitary adenoma in the literature at the time of analysis, Cossu et al. noted that the mean age of patients with mixed gangliocytoma/pituitary adenoma at presentation was 44.5 years with 80% of the cases having presented in females [13]. The youngest patient reported in the series was 16 years of age [13].

Based on imaging studies, Cossu and colleagues noted that in the 71 cases in which information was available, 18 tumors (25%) were located in the sella only, 23 (32%) cases demonstrated some evidence of suprasellar extension, 30 cases (42%) showed evidence of either cavernous or sphenoid sinus invasion, and 1 case (1.4%) appeared to be more widely invasive [13]. In mixed tumors, distinction of the gangliocytoma component from the adenoma component is often not possible. Tumors have been described as showing homogeneous enhancement after contrast [14, 15]. On T1-weighted magnetic resonance images (MRI), tumors may be variously hyperintense, hypointense or mixed iso- and hypointense [14, 15]. On T2-weighted images, tumors may be either mixed iso- and hyperintense or hyperintense [14, 15].

PATHOLOGY

The two components of the tumor comprise variable proportions of the neoplasm. The adenoma component is typically composed of a relatively monomorphic population of rounded epithelioid cells arranged in a sheet-like configuration (Figure 1).

The cells may have eosinophilic or relatively clear cytoplasm with oval nuclei. The interface between both components of the mixed tumor may be quite distinct microscopically (Figure 2).

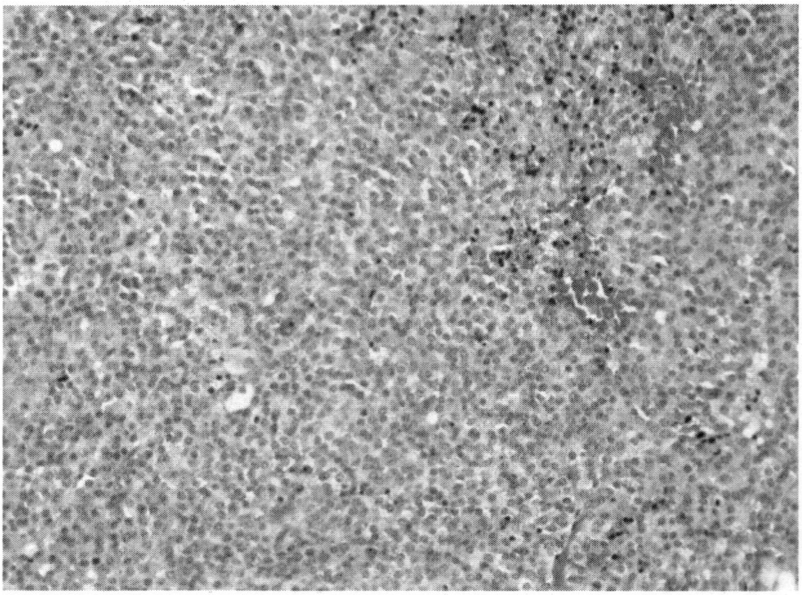

Figure 1. A pituitary adenoma arising in the adenohypophysis marked by a monomorphic proliferation of rounded cells (hematoxylin and eosin, original magnification 200X).

The gangliocytomatous component of the tumor is marked by increased number of large neuronal or ganglionic cells arranged against a neuropil-like background (Figure 3). The background is not particularly hypercellular and lacks an atypical proliferation of glial cells, suggestive of a ganglioglioma. The neuronal cells may be irregularly grouped or clustered and are not necessarily evenly distributed throughout the lesion. Dysplastic features may be present including cytomegaly, multipolarity, multinucleation, and abnormal Nissl substance distribution (Figure 4). Mitotic figures are not typically present.

In some mixed lesions, isolated ganglionic cells may be seen within the adenomatous component of the tumor (Figure 5).

The adenomatous component of the tumor is well known to stain with synaptophysin antibody. Focal chromogranin immunoreactivity may also be encountered. In contrast to normal anterior pituitary gland tissue, adenomas show loss of the normal nested architectural pattern of cells; this can be highlighted with a reticulin stain, if needed. Adenomas that are hormonally productive may stain with antibodies directed at the hormone being produced. Some of the adenomas seen in these mixed tumors appear to be hormonally inactive. As previously discussed, tumors that have been described to be hormonally active have produced growth hormone, prolactin and adrenocorticotrophic hormone (Figure 6). Pit-1 immunoreactivity has also been reported in the adenomatous component of these tumors [21].

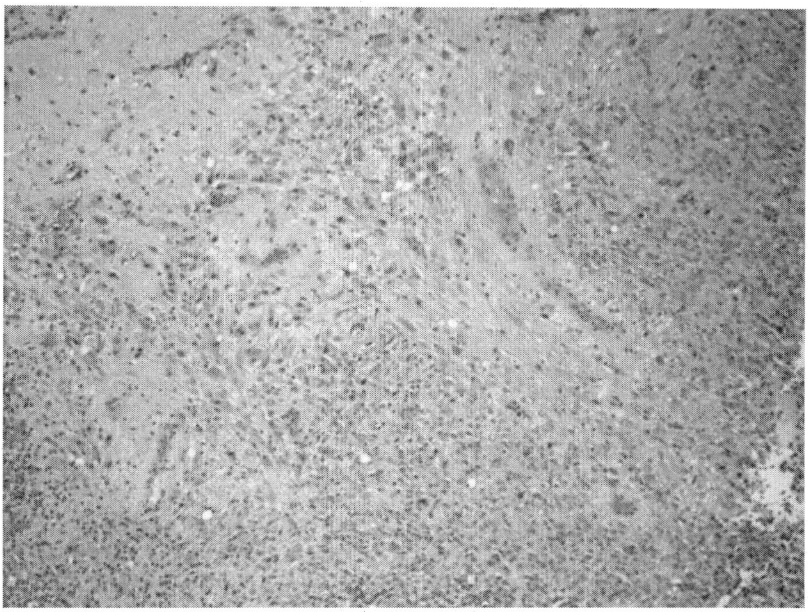

Figure 2. At the interface between a pituitary adenoma (bottom) and a gangliocytoma (top) (hematoxylin and eosin, original magnification 100X).

The gangliocytoma component of the tumor may variably express immunostaining with antibodies to NeuN, neurofilament, synaptophysin and MAP 2 [21, 22]. The background neuropil-like stroma does not stain with glial fibrillary acidic protein (GFAP) [21]. Interestingly, Pit-1 expression has been described in some cases in the ganglionic cells [21]. The ganglionic cells do not stain with the pituitary hormone stains. Asa et al. observed that the ganglionic cells may also express hypothalamic hormones such as somatostatin, gonadotropin-releasing hormone, corticotropin-releasing hormone, and growth hormone-releasing hormone. [23]. Cell proliferation indices, using antibodies such as MIB-1 or Ki-67, have been anecdotally reported as low [11, 15]. Chen and coworkers examined two tumors with MIB-1 antibody and noted indices in both tumors of <1%. [11]. In a series of 20 tumors, Yang et al. reported a Ki-67 labeling index of less than 5% in all cases [15].

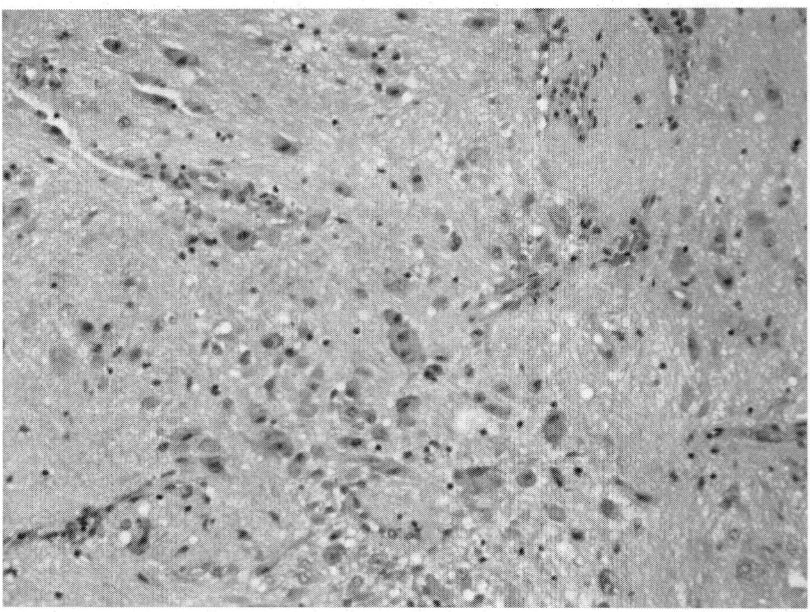

Figure 3. A geographically distinct area of the tumor resembling a gangliocytoma, marked by scattered neurons/ganglion cells arranged against a fibrillary background (hematoxylin and eosin, original magnification 200X).

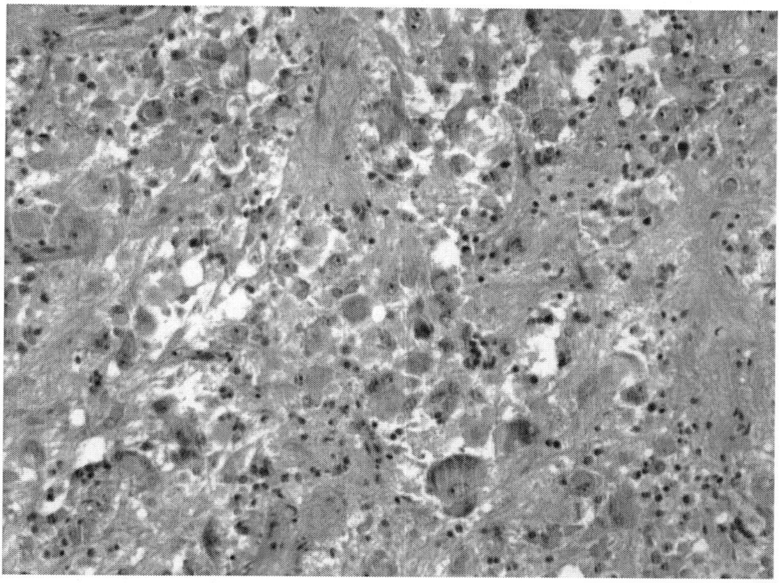

Figure 4. Atypical neuronal cells may be seen and may include neuronal cytomegaly and abnormal Nissl substance distribution (hematoxylin and eosin, original magnification 200X).

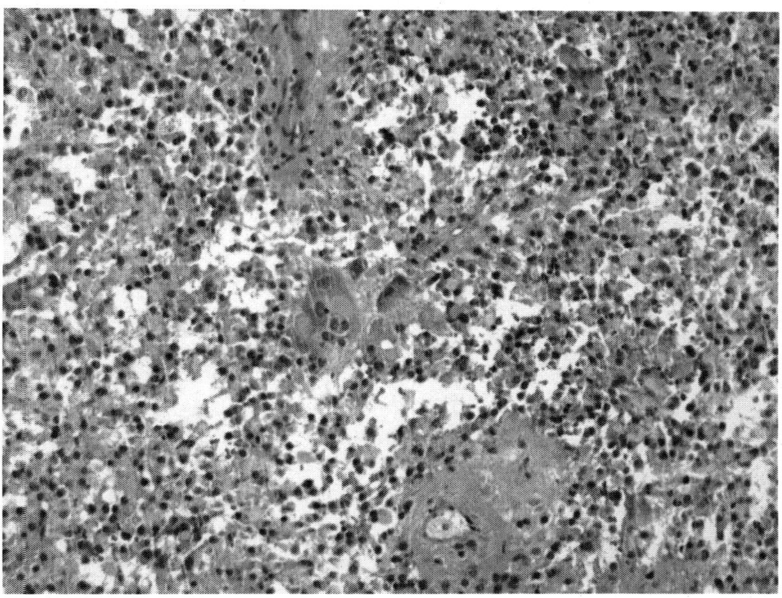

Figure 5. Sometimes, isolated ganglionic cells may be intermixed in the adenomatous component (hematoxylin and eosin, original magnification 200X).

Differential Diagnosis

The differential diagnostic consideration are more of an imaging issue than a pathology one. There are a number of tumors that can arise in the pituitary gland that can resemble a circumscribed mixed gangliocytoma/pituitary adenoma including pituicytoma, granular cell tumor, spindle cell oncocytoma, craniopharyngioma, and meningioma. Morphologically, none of these entities resembles the gangliocytoma-pituitary adenoma. Of note, rare cases of ganglioglioma of the adenohypophysis have been described, which may resemble the gangliocytomatous component [24-26]. Gangliogliomas are histologically marked by the presence of a glioma-like component intermixed with the atypical neuronal component. A rare case of a 54-year-old woman with a growth hormone secreting pituitary adenoma admixed with both a ganglioglioma and gangliocytoma was reported by Jukes and coworkers in 2016 [27].

Treatment

The management of these mixed tumors is similar to that employed for pituitary adenomas. Functional tumors may be medically managed. Surgery is employed for tumors that are symptomatic because of size or hormone production. Most cases are usually approached transsphenoidally; although reports of transcranial or combined approached have been documented [13]. In the 37 cases of mixed adenoma-gangliocytoma reported by Cossu et al., 30 cases achieved postoperative hormonal normalization with 13 of those cases having undergone a complete resection [13]. Occasionally, radiotherapy or chemotherapy has been employed in the management of tumors but the number of such treated cases is too small to be certain how beneficial these approaches were [13, 28].

HISTOGENESIS

According to the literature, there have been three different hypotheses proposed to explain the origin of these tumors [6, 14, 21, 29, 30]. One thought is that one starts with a gangliocytoma or displaced hypothalamic neurons, the presence of which induces an adenoma via paracrine secretion of hypothalamic hormones. Another proposed theory suggests that the ganglionic component originates from neuronal differentiation within the adenoma component of the tumor by a process referred to as transdifferentiation. Lastly, it has been suggested that both the adenoma and gangliocytoma components of the tumor may share a common origin from a progenitor or stem cell located in the adenohypophysis of the pituitary gland that has the capability to differentiate in either or both directions.

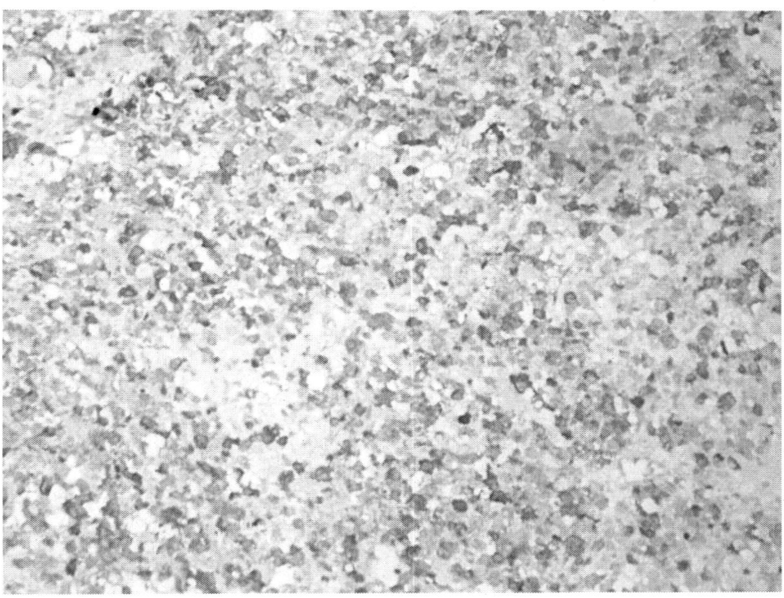

Figure 6. Immunostaining with antibody to growth hormone shows positive staining in the adenoma (original magnification 200X).

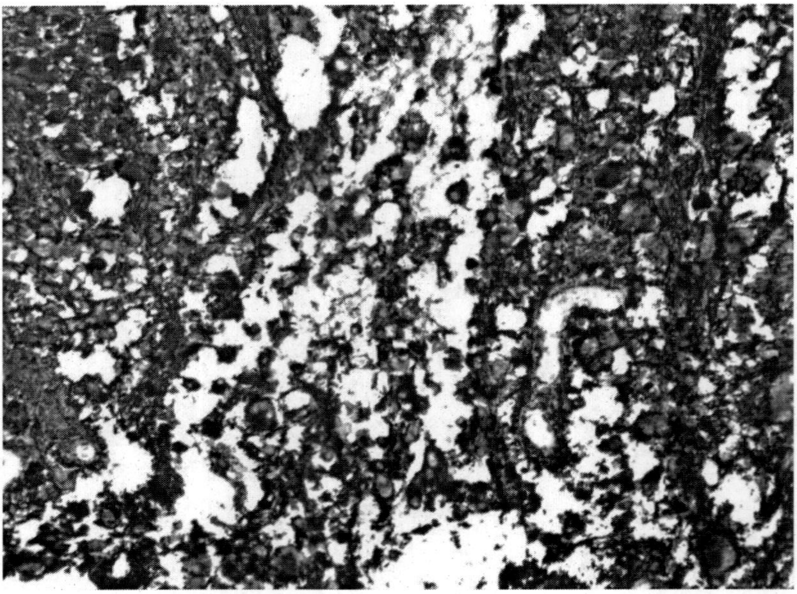

Figure 7. Synaptophysin immunoreactivity was observed both in the cells of the adenoma as well as the larger neuronal cells on the gangliocytoma (original magnification 200X).

REFERENCES

[1] Capper D, Becker AJ, Giannini C, Figarella-Branger D, Huse JT, Rosenblum MK, Blümcke I, Wiestler OD. Gangliocytoma. In: *WHO Classification of Tumours of the Central Nervous System* (Editors: Louis DN, Ohgaki H, Wiestler OD, Cavenee WK, Ellison DW, Figarella-Branger D, Perry A, Reifenberger G, von Deimling A). IARC. Lyon, FR, 2016. pp. 136-137.

[2] Thom M, Blümcke I, Aronica E. Long-term epilepsy-associated tumors. *Brain Pathol.,* 2012; 22(3): 350-379.

[3] Eng C, Murday V, Seal S, Mohammed S, Hodgson SV, Chaudary MA, Fentiman IS, Ponder BA, Eeles RA. Cowden syndrome and Lhermitte-Duclos disease in a family: a single genetic syndrome with pleiotropy? *J. Med. Genet.,* 1994; 31(6): 458-461.

[4] Vital A, Vital C, Martin-Negrier ML, McGrogan G, Bioulac P, Trojani M, Loiseau H, Rougier A. Lhermitte-Duclos type cerebellum hamartoma and Cowden disease. *Clin. Neuropathol.,* 1994; 13(4): 229-231.

[5] Eberhart CG, Wiestler OD, Eng C. Dysplastic cerebellar gangliocytoma (Lhermitte-Duclos disease). In: *WHO Classification of Tumours of the Central Nervous System* (Editors: Louis DN, Ohgaki H, Wiestler OD, Cavenee WK, Ellison DW, Figarella-Branger D, Perry A, Reifenberger G, von Deimling A). IARC. Lyon, FR, 2016. pp. 142-143.

[6] Horvath E, Kovacs K, Scheithauer BW, Lloyd RV, Smyth HS. Pituitary adenoma with neuronal choristoma (PANCH): composite lesion or lineage infidelity? *Ultrastruct. Pathol.,* 1994; 18: 565-574.

[7] Saeger W, Lüdecke DK, Buchfelder M, Fahlbusch R, Quabbe H-J, Petersenn S. Pathohistological classification of pituitary tumors: 10 years of experience with the German Pituitary Tumor Registry. *European J. Endocrinol.,* 2007; 156: 203-216.

[8] Puchner MJ, Lüdecke DK, Saeger W, Riedel M, Asa SL. Gangliocytomas of the sellar region - a review. *Exp. Clin. Endocrinol. Diabetes,* 1995; 103: 129-149.

[9] Geddes JF, Jansen GH, Robinson SF, Gömri E, Holton JL, Monson JP, Besser GM, Révész T. 'Gangliocytomas' of the pituitary: a heterogeneous group of lesions with differing histogenesis *Am. J. Surg. Pathol.,* 2000; 24: 607-613.

[10] Towfighi J, Salam MM, McLendon RE, Powers S, Page RB. Ganglion cell-containing tumors of the pituitary gland. *Arch. Pathol. Lab. Med.,* 1996; 120: 369-377.

[11] Chen A, Xu J, Zhong P, Huang X, Xu M. Pituitary adenoma with gangliocytoma: Report of two cases. *Oncol. Let.,* 2014; 8: 781-784.

[12] Kurosaki M, Saeger W, Lüdecke DK. Intrasellar gangliocytomas associated with acromegaly. *Brain Tumor Pathol.,* 2002; 19: 63-67.

[13] Cossu G, Daniel RT, Messerer M. Gangliocytomas of the sellar region: A challenging diagnosis. *Clin. Neurol. Neurosurg.,* 2016; 149: 122-135.

[14] Qiao N, Ye Z, Wang Y, Li S, Mao Y, Bao W, Che X, Qin Z, Xu W, Shen M, Chen H, Shou X, Zhao Y. Gangliocytomas in the sellar region. *Clin. Neurol. Neurosurg.,* 2014; 126: 156-161.

[15] Yang B, Yang C, Sun Y, Du J, Liu P, Jia G, Zhang Y, Wang J, Xu Y, Wang S. Mixed gangliocytoma-pituitary adenoma in the sellar region: a large-scale single-center experience. *Acta Neurochir.,* 2018; 160: 1989-1999.

[16] Li Y, Racadot O, Kujas M, Kovardri M, Pellon F, Racadot J. Immunocytochemistry of four mixed pituitary adenomas and intrasellar gangliocytomas associated with different clinical syndromes: acromegaly, amenorrhea-galactorrhea, Cushing's disease and isolated tumoral syndrome. *Acta Neuropathol.,* 1989; 77(3): 320-328.

[17] Saeger W, Puchner MJ, Lüdecke DK. Combined sellar gangliocytoma and pituitary adenoma in acromegaly or Cushing's disease. A report of three cases. *Virchows Arch.,* 1994; 425: 93-99.

[18] Mikami S, Kameyama K, Takahashi S Yoshida K, Kawase T, Sano T, Mukai M. Combined gangliocytoma and prolactinoma of the pituitary gland. *Endocr. Pathol.,* 2008; 19(2): 117-121.

[19] Puchner MJ, Lüdecke DK, Valdueza JM, Saeger, Willig RP, Stalla GK, Odink RJ. Cushing's disease in a child caused by corticotropin-releasing hormone-secreting intrasellar gangliocytoma associated with an adrenocorticotropic hormone-secreting pituitary adenoma. *Neurosurgery,* 1993; 33(5): 920-924.

[20] Kissiedu JO, Prayson RA. Sellar gangliocytoma with adrenocorticotropic and prolactin adenoma. *J. Clin. Neurosci.,* 2016; 24: 141-142.

[21] Lopes MBS, Sloan E, Polder J. Mixed gangliocytoma-pituitary adenoma. Insights on the pathogenesis of a rare sellar tumor. *Am. J. Surg. Pathol.,* 2017; 41: 586-595.

[22] Kontogeorgos G, Mourouti G, Kyrodimou E, Liapi-Avgeri G, Parisi E. Ganglion cell containing pituitary adenomas: signs of neuronal differentiation in adenoma cells. *Acta Neuropathol.,* 2006; 112: 21-28.

[23] Asa SL, Scheithauer BW, Bilbao JM, Horvath E, Ryan N, Kovacs K, Randall RV, Laws ER Jr, Singer W, Linfoot JA, Thorne MO, Vale W. A case for hypothalamic acromegaly: a clinicopathological study of six patients with hypothalamic gangliocytomas producing growth hormone-releasing factor. *J. Clin. Endocrinol. Metab.,* 1984; 58(5): 796-803.

[24] Hong Y, Fang Y, We Q, Zhang J, Wang Y. Ganglioglioma of the adenohypophysis mimicking pituitary adenoma. *Medicine,* 2018; http://dx.doi.org/10.1097/MD.0000000000011583.

[25] Jalali R, Deopujari CE, Bhutani R, Suhas U, Raiasekharan P, Kane SV, Gupta T. Suprasellar ganglioglioma with unusual diffuse involvement of the entire optico-chiasmal hypothalamic pathway. *J. Cancer Res. Ther.,* 2008; 4(3): 140-143.

[26] Scheithauer BW, Silva AI, Parisi JE, Kovacs K, Horvath E. Ganglioglioma of the neurohypophysis. *Endocr. Pathol.,* 2008: 19(2): 112-116.

[27] Jukes A, Allan R, Rawson R, Buckland ME. Growth hormone secreting pituitary adenoma with admixed gangliocytoma and ganglioglioma. *J. Clin. Neurosci.,* 2016; 31: 202-204.

[28] Yano S Hide T, Uekawa K, Honda Y, Mikami Y, Kuratsu JI. Mixed pituitary gangliocytoma and prolactinoma resistant to the cabergoline treatment. *World Neurosurg.,* 95: 620 e617-620, e622.

[29] Chen J, Hersmus N, Van Duppen V, Caesens P, Denef C, Vankelecom H. The adult pituitary contains a cell population displaying stem/progenitor cell and early embryonic characteristics. *Endocrinology,* 2005; 146: 3985-3998.

[30] Vidal S, Horvath E, Kovacs K, Lloyd RV, Smyth HS. Reversible transdifferentiation: interconversion of somatotrophs and lactotrophs in pituitary hyperplasia. *Mod. Pathol.,* 2001; 14: 20-28.

In: The Pituitary Gland and Adrenal Glands ISBN: 978-1-53617-605-6
Editor: Noémi Barta

Chapter 4

GRANULAR CELL TUMOR OF THE PITUITARY GLAND

Richard A. Prayson*[1,*], *MD, MEd
and Elizabeth E. O'Toole*[2], *MD
Cleveland Clinic[1] and MetroHealth Medical Center[2],
Cleveland, OH, US

ABSTRACT

Granular tumors are relatively rare neoplasms that most commonly arise in the neurohypophysis or posterior portion of the pituitary gland. Most present in adults, with a peak incidence in the 5th and 6th decades of life, and they are more frequently encountered in women. These tumors most commonly present with visual field defects secondary to compression of the optic chiasm. The lesion is typically well circumscribed and lobulated. The lesion is marked by a proliferation of large polygonal or slightly elongated cells which contain abundant granular eosinophilic cytoplasm, as its name suggests. The granular quality of the cytoplasm is due to the large number of phagolysosomes that fill it. Immunophenotypically, granular cell tumors, like pituicytomas and spindle cell oncocytomas, are characterized by strong nuclear

* Corresponding Author's E-mail: praysor@ccf.org.

staining with antibody to thyroid transcription factor-1, suggesting that the tumor is derived from pituicytes in the neurohypophysis. Granular cell tumors are generally considered benign tumors and surgical resection is the treatment of choice for larger and symptomatic lesions. This chapter will review the clinicopathologic features of this neoplasm and include a discussion of differential diagnosis.

INTRODUCTION

In 1893, Boyce and Beadles, in a study of the pathology of the pituitary gland, described a case in which they observed cells with granular cytoplasm forming a small tumor about a quarter of an inch in diameter in the neurohypophysis [1]. The tumor was reported to be an incidental finding in an autopsy in a patient who had senile dementia. This has been purported by many to be the first description of a granular cell tumor of the pituitary gland. In 1921, Sternberg described similar findings and coined the term "hypophyseal choristoma" for the tumor [2]. He conjectured that the lesion was of glial origin. In 1955, Luse and Kernohan examined 1364 pituitary glands obtained at autopsy over a 30 year period of time [3]. In 88 cases (6.45%), they noted small tumor-like nodules of large granular cells; in three cases, multiple nodules were noted in a single gland. A few years earlier, von Luthy and Klinger described a case of a symptomatic tumor in a patient with visual symptoms secondary to compression of the optic chiasm [4]. This established the idea that these lesions could grow in size over time, particularly in middle-aged to older adults. In subsequent years, similar tumors were reported under a variety of other names including myoblastoma, pituicytoma, Abrikossoff tumor, granular cell neuroma, and tumor of granular cell [5]. Although the origin of these tumors is still a matter of some debate, the general thought is that they arise from pituicytes in the neurohypophysis. Given their immunoreactivity with antibody to thyroid transcription factor-1 (TTF-1), they are now thought to be on the spectrum with other tumors that also arise in the posterior pituitary gland (pituicytomas and spindle cell oncocytomas), which are also presumably derived from pituicytes [6].

Clinical Presentation

While the majority of granular cell tumors of the pituitary have been described to arise in adults, anecdotal cases have been documented in children [7]. There appears to be a female predominance to cases that have been reported with a peak incidence in the fifth and sixth decades of life [6]. The lesion may appear as small incidental microscopic clusters of cells that have been referred to as tumourlets or tumourettes [8, 3] and less commonly as larger, symptomatic masses. In one of the more recent autopsy series which systematically looked for incidental tumors, Tomita and Gates found granular cell tumors in nine of the 100 glands examined (9%) [9]. Interestingly, three of the cases had coexistent adenomas. Fourteen additional cases in the series showed small granular cell nests. Tumors typically are found in the neurohypophysis or posterior pituitary gland or the pituitary stalk/infundibulum.

The most common presentation for symptomatic tumors includes visual field defects, related to compression of the optic chiasm by the tumor [10]. A variety of other presentations have been less frequently encountered and include symptoms related to anterior pituitary gland dysfunction (galactorrhea, amenorrhea, decreased libido and panhypopituitarism) and neuropsychological changes. Rare instances of diabetes insipidus have been documented [10]. As previously mentioned [9], occasional tumors may be associated with concomitant pituitary adenomas [9-12]. In one meta-analysis of the literature reviewing the findings in 64 tumors, the most common presentations included visual disturbances (64.1%), headaches (32.8%), amenorrhea (18.8%) and fatigue (10.9%) [13].

Imaging studies usually show features of a circumscribed mass that may be either homogenously or heterogenously contrast enhancing on magnetic resonance imaging (MRI) studies [13-15]. The findings are not specific enough to make a diagnosis. Calcifications are not generally observed in granular cell tumors; this can potentially be helpful in distinguishing a granular cell tumor from a sellar or suprasellar craniopharyngioma, which is often calcified. The lack of a dural attachment would allow for distinction of a granular cell tumor from a meningioma.

PATHOLOGY

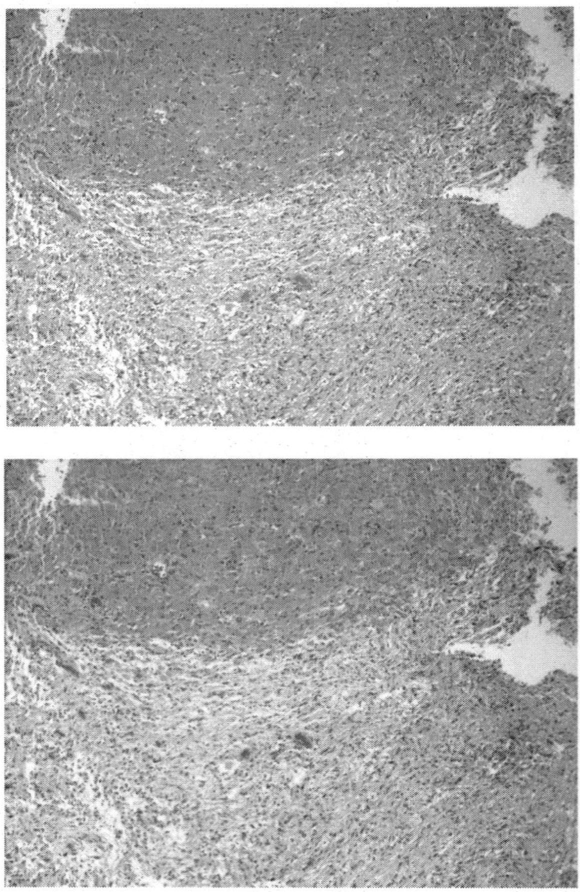

Figure 1. Low magnification appearance of a granular cell tumor (top) arising in the neurohypophysis of the pituitary gland (bottom). The tumor appears circumscribed and nonencapsulated (hematoxylin and eosin, original magnification 100X).

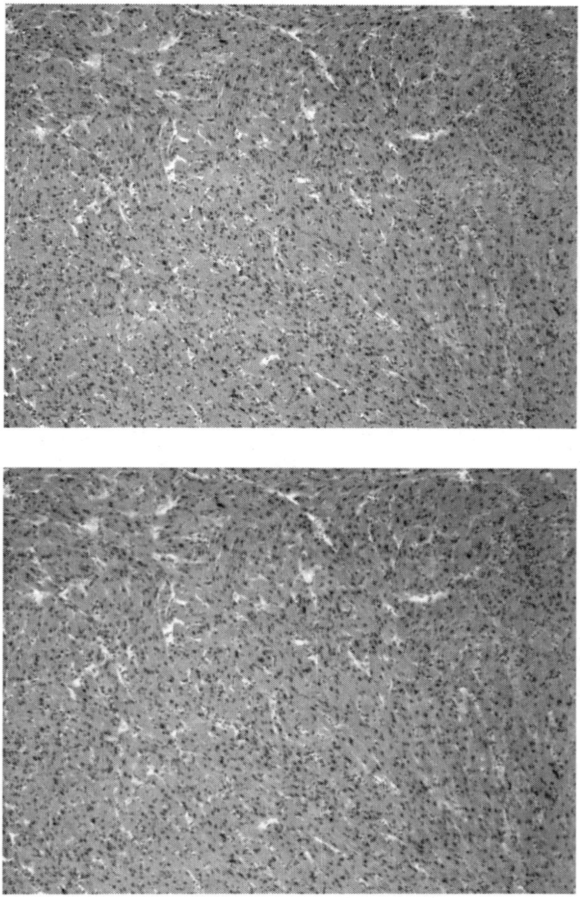

Figure 2. Cells in a granular cell tumor are typically rounded to slightly elongated in configuration (hematoxylin and eosin, original magnification 200X).

Grossly, tumors are well circumscribed, nonencapsulated and lobulated (Figure 1). They have a soft and rubbery consistency and overall are firmer in consistency than pituitary adenomas [6]. They only rarely are known to invade surrounding structures such as the optic chiasm or hypothalamus. Cystic changes, necrosis, and hemorrhage are unusual findings grossly.

Microscopically, similar to their counterparts in other parts of the bodies, granular cell tumors are marked by a proliferation of tumor cells which are generally rounded/polygonal or slightly elongated with abundant cytoplasm (Figure 2). Tumor cells may be arranged in nodules, sheets or in fascicular patterns. The cytoplasm of tumor cells is filled with eosinophilic granules which correspond to large phagolysosomes on ultrastructural examination (Figure 3) [16-18]. Tumor cell nuclei are small and lack prominent nucleoli. Perivascular lymphocytes may be occasionally encountered in tumors (Figure 4).

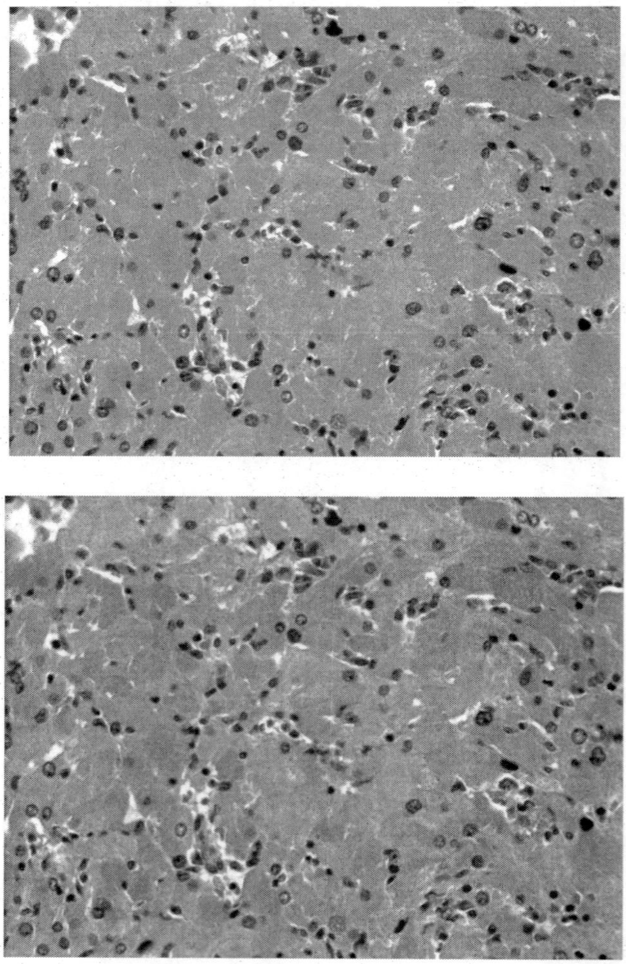

Figure 3. The cytoplasm is marked by a granular quality due to large atypical lysosomes (hematoxylin and eosin, original magnification 400X).

Occasional tumors may demonstrate some evidence of nuclear pleomorphism, multinucleated cells, prominent nucleolation or increased mitotic activity [19, 20]; such tumors have been referred to as atypical granular cell tumors. The significance of such changes remains uncertain.

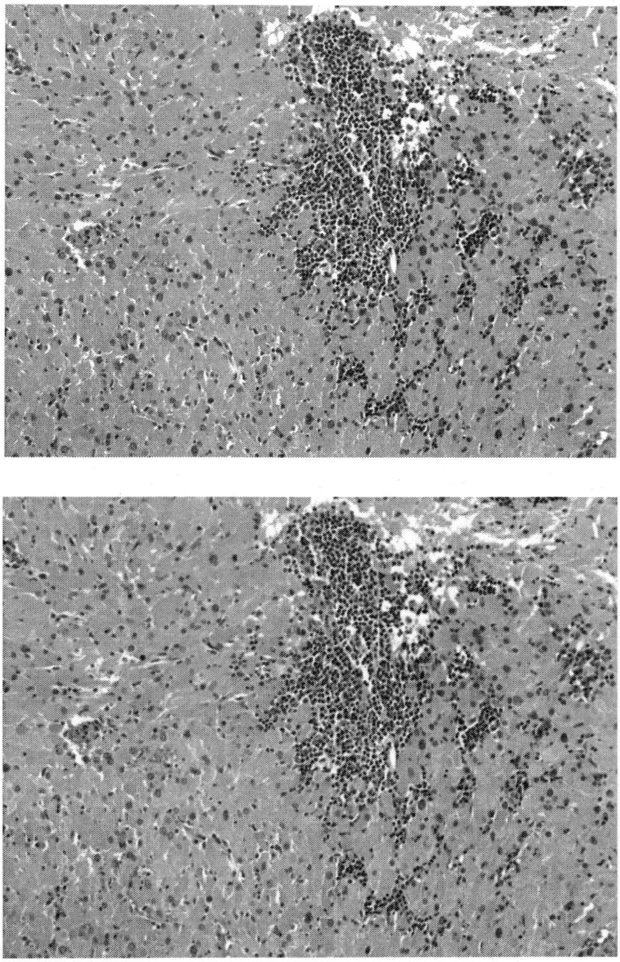

Figure 4. Focally, benign appearing lymphocytes may be intermixed in the tumor (hematoxylin and eosin, original magnification 200X).

Granular cell tumors are well known to stain with antibodies to S-100 protein (Figure 5), CD68, alpha-1-antitrypsin, epithelial membrane antigen (EMA), vimentin, cathepsin B and alpha-1-antichymotrypsin [6]. They do not stain with pituitary hormones or other markers that stain pituitary adenomas (such as synaptophysin, cytokeratins). Variable immunoreactivity to GFAP antibody can be seen. As previously mentioned, nuclear staining with TTF-1 has been more recently recognized (Figure 6) [21, 22].

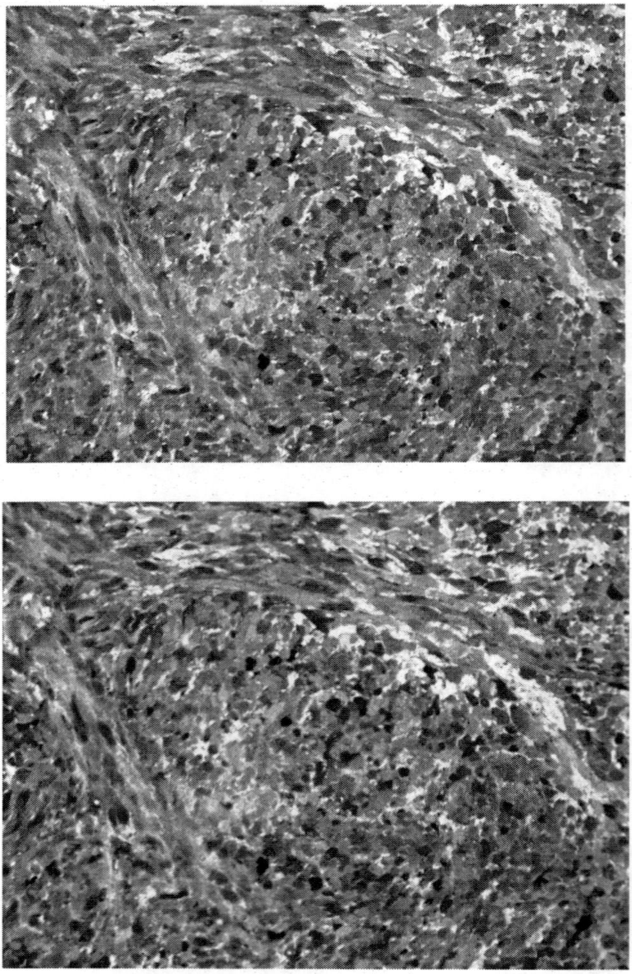

Figure 5. Diffuse strong S-100 protein immunoreactivity in a granular cell tumor (original magnification 200X).

Molecular and genetic data on these tumors is sparse. Mete et al., in a study of 3 granular cell tumors, noted no evidence of BRAF V600E mutations or BRAF-KIAA fusion in these three tumors [22]. Similarly,

BRAF alterations were also not noted in the seven spindle cell oncocytomas and four pituicytomas which were also evaluated in this study [22]. IDH-1 (R132H) mutations by immunohistochemical staining were also not observed in the granular cell tumors [22].

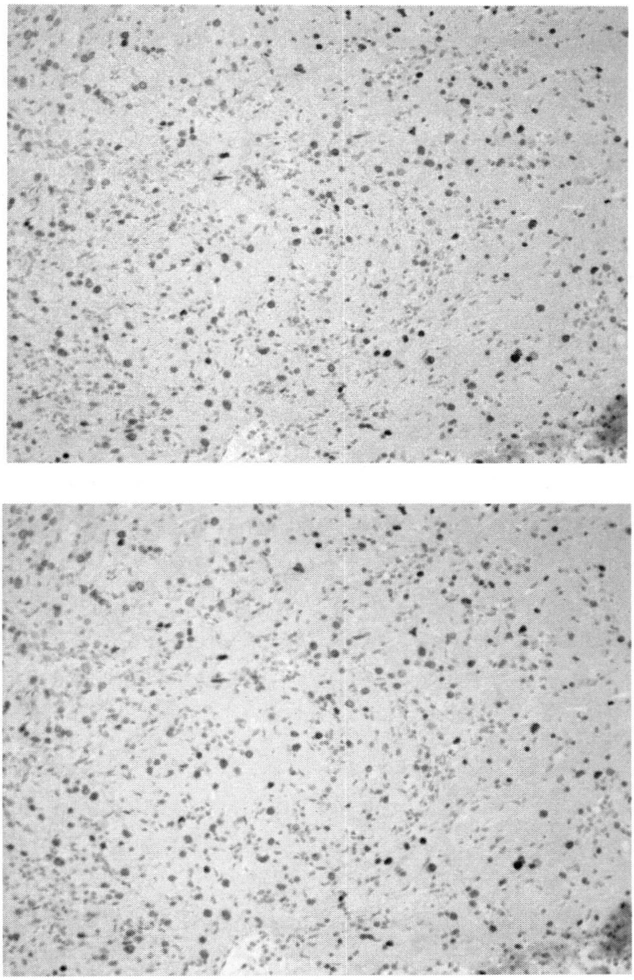

Figure 6. Nuclear immunoreactivity in a granular cell tumor with antibody to thyroid transcription factor-1 (TTF-1) (original magnification 200X).

DIFFERENTIAL DIAGNOSIS

Due to their location and the radiographic appearance of a circumscribed mass, granular cell tumors may be confused with pituitary adenomas. Morphologically, granular cell tumor cells typically have more cytoplasm and the granular quality of the cytoplasm is not a feature observed in adenomas. Granular cell tumors also do not stain with immunomarkers observed in adenomas including synaptophysin, cytokeratin, and pituitary hormones (i.e., adrenocorticotropic hormone (ACTH), growth hormone (GH), follicle-stimulating hormone (FSH), luteinizing hormone (LH), prolactin (PL), and thyroid stimulating hormone (TSH). TTF-1 immunoreactivity is not seen in adenomas.

Meningiomas and craniopharyngiomas are two other low grade, circumscribed neoplasms that arise frequently in that location that on imaging can mimic granular cell tumor. Meningiomas are usually dural based, lack the abundant granular cytoplasm, do not stain with TTF-1 and do stain with markers such as progesterone receptor (PR) and somatostatin receptor 2a (SSTR2a). Craniopharyngiomas are morphologically very distinct from granular cell tumors with their epithelial appearance, stellate reticulum, basal palisading cells and wet keratin.

Distinction of the granular cell tumor from spindle cell oncocytomas and pituicytomas is, at times, more challenging. It is recognized that all of these tumors stain with TTF-1 antibody. Pituicytomas are classically marked by more elongated cells arranged in fascicles or in a storiform pattern [23]. The cytoplasmic granularity of the cells in a granular cell tumor are generally absent in a pituicytoma. Spindle cell oncocytoma is characterized by interlacing fascicles of spindled cells with eosinophilic cytoplasm [24]. The cytoplasm is variably oncocytic to clear but generally lacks the granularity of the granular cell tumor.

Rarely, granular cell tumors have been described arising in other areas in the central nervous system including the spinal meninges, third ventricle region and cranial meninges [25-27]. Also of note, one of the variants of an astrocytoma is marked by the presence of granular cells, identical to those seen in a granular cell tumor [28]; in some of these tumors, focal areas of essentially confluent granular cells with little if any recognizable astrocytoma component may be encountered.

Treatment and Prognosis

In the World Health Organization (WHO) classification of brain tumors, granular cell tumors of the pituitary have been designated as grade I neoplasms [6]. They are considered clinically benign tumors with slow progression and a lack of an infiltrative growth pattern [10, 16, 17]. Surgical excision is the treatment of choice for symptomatic or large tumors. There is no need for adjuvant radiation therapy or chemotherapy. Postoperative sequelae may include hypopituitarism and persistent diabetes insipidus [10].

References

[1] Boyce R, Beadles CF. A further contribution to the study of the pathology of the hypophysis cerebri. *J. Pathol. Bacteriol.*, 1893; 1: 359-383.

[2] Sternberg C. Ein choristoma der neurohypophyse bei ausgebreitetenoedemen [A choristoma of the neurohypophysis in spreading edema]. *Zbl. Allg. Path. Anat.,* 1921; 31: 585-591.

[3] Luse SA, Kernohan JW. Granular cell tumors of the stalk and posterior lobe of the pituitary gland. *Cancer*, 1955; 8(3): 616-622.

[4] von Luthy F, Klinger M. Der tumorettentumor des hypophysenhinterlappens [The tumor tumor of hypophyseal lobe]. *Schweiz. Z. Allg. Path.,* 1951; 14: 721-729.

[5] Vaquero J, Leunda G, Cabezudo JM, Salazar AR, de Miguel J. Granular pituicytomas of the pituitary stalk. *Acta Neurchirurgica,* 1981; 59: 209-215.

[6] Fuller GN, Brat SJ, Wesseling P, Roncaroli F. Granular cell tumour of the sellar region. In: *WHO Classification of Tumours of the Central Nervous System.* (Louis DN, Ohgaki H, Wiestler OD, Cavenee WK, Ellison DW, Gigarella-Branger D, Perry A, Reofenberger G, von Deimling A). IARC. Lyon, FR. 201. Pp. 329-331.

[7] Benites Filho PR, Sakamoto D, Machuca TN, Sarapiao MJ, Ditzel L, Bieggi Torres LF. Granular cell tumor of the neurohypophysis: report of a case with unusual age presentation. *Virchows Arch.,* 2005; 447(3): 649-652.

[8] Shanklin WM. The origin, histology and senescence of tumourettes in the human neurohypophysis. *Acta Anat. (Basel),* 1953; 18(1): 1-20.

[9] Tomita T, Gates E. Pituitary adenomas and granular cell tumors. Incidence, cell type, and location of tumor in 100 pituitary glands at autopsy. *Am. J. Clin. Pathol.,* 1999; 111(6): 817-825.

[10] Cohen-Gadol AA, Pichelmann MA, Link MJ, Scheithauer BW, Krecke KN, Young WF Jr, Giannini C. Granular cell tumor of the sellar and suprasellar region: clinicopathologic study of 11 cases and literature review. *Mayo Clin. Proc.,* 2003; 78(5): 567-573.

[11] Barrande G, Kujas M, Gancel A, Turpic G, Bruckert E, Kuhn JM, Luton JP. Granular cell tumors. Rare tumors of the neurohypophysis. *Presse Med.,* 1995; 24(30): 1376-1380.

[12] Losa M, Saeger W, Mortini P, Pandolfi C, Terreni MR, Taccagni G, Giovanelli M. Acromegaly associated with a granular cell tumor of the neurophypophysis: a clinical and histological study. Case report. *J. Neurosurg.,* 2000; 93(1): 121-126.

[13] Covington MF, Chin SS, Osborn AG. Pituicytoma, spindle cell oncocytoma and granular cell tumor: Clarification and meta-analysis of the world literature since 1983. *Am. J. Neuroradioll,* 2011; 32: 2067-2011.

[14] Park SJ, Chang YH, Yang NR, Seo EK. Granular cell tumor in the pituitary stalk: A case report. *Brain Tumor Res. Treat.,* 2015; 3(1): 60-63.

[15] Han F, Gao L, Wang Y, Jin Y, Lv Y, Yao Z, Zhang J. Clinical and imaging features of granular cell tumor of the neurohypophysis. A retrospective analysis. *Medicine,* 2018; 97: 9(e9745).

[16] Liwnicz BH, Liwnicz RG, Huff JS, McBride BHG, Tew JM Jr. Giant granular cell tumor of the suprasellar area: immunocytochemical and electron microscopic studies. *Neurosurgery*, 1984; 15: 246-251.

[17] Schaller BM, Kirsch E, Tolnay M, Mindermann T. Symptomatic granular cell tumor of the pituitary gland: case report and review f the literature. *Neurosurgery,* 1998; 42: 166-171.

[18] Vinores SA. Demonstration of glial fibrillary acidic (GFA) protein by electron microscopy in the granular cells of a choristoma of the neurohypophysis. *Histochemistry,* 1991; 96: 265-269.

[19] Kasashima S, Oda Y, Nozaki J, Shirasaki M, Nakanishi I. A case of atypical granular cell tumor of the neurohypophysis. *Pathol. Int.,* 2000; 50(7): 568-573.

[20] Vogelgesang S, Junge MH, Pahnke J, Gaab MR, Warzok RW. Sellar/suprasellar mass in a 59-year-old woman. *Brain Pathol.,* 2002; 12(1): 135-136.

[21] Lee EB, Tihan T, Scheithauer BW, Zhang PJ, Gonatas NK. Thyroid transcription factor 1 expression in sellar tumors: a histogenetic marker? *J. Neuropathol. Exp. Neurol.,* 2009; 68(5): 482-488.

[22] Mete O, Lopes MB, Asa SL. Spindle cell oncocytomas and granular cell tumors of the pituitary are variants of pituicytomas. *Am. J. Surg. Pathol.,* 2013; 37(11): 1694-1699.

[23] Brat DJ, Scheithauer BW, Staugaitis SM, Holtzman RN, Morgello S, Burger PC. Pituicytomas: a distinctive low-grade glioma of the neurohypophysis. *Am. J. Surg. Pathol.,* 2000; 24(3): 362-368.

[24] Roncaroli F, Scheithauer BW, Cenacchi G, Horvath K, Kovacs K, Lloyd RV, Abell-Aleff P, Santi M, Yates AJ. 'Spindle cell oncocytoma' of the adenohypophysis: a tumor of folliculostellate cells? *Am. J. Surg. Pathol.,* 2002; 26(8): 1048-1055.

[25] Vaghasiya VL, Nasit JG, Parikh PA, Trivedi PP. Intradural spinal granular cell tumor. *Asian J. Neurosurg.,* 2014; 9(2): 96-98.

[26] Vang R, Heck K, Fuller GN, Medeiros LJ. Granular cell tumor of intracranial meninges. *Clin. Neuropathol.*, 2000; 19(1): 41-44.

[27] Ulrich J, Heitz PU, Fischer T, Obrist E, Gullotta F. Granular cell tumors: evidence for heterogenous tumor cell differentiation. An immunocytochemical study. *Virchows Arch. B Cell Pathol. Incl. Mol. Pathol.*, 1987; 53(1): 557.

[28] Schittenhelm J, Psasas T. Glioblastoma with granular cell astrocytoma features: A case report and review of the literature. *Clin. Neuropathol.*, 2010; 29(5): 323-329.

In: The Pituitary Gland and Adrenal Glands ISBN: 978-1-53617-605-6
Editor: Noémi Barta

Chapter 5

THE ADRENAL GLANDS: FUNCTION, REGULATION AND DISORDERS

Levent Soydan**, MD
Department of Radiology, Haydarpasa Numune Research and Training Hospital, Istanbul, Turkey

ABSTRACT

The adrenal glands are paired structures located superior to the kidneys in the retroperitoneal space. Mineralocorticoids, glucocorticoids and adrenal androgens are synthesized respectively in the zona glomerulosa, zona fasciculatis and zona reticularisthat make up the cortex, while the inner adrenal medulla produces the catecholamines and peptides. Aldosterone, the main mineralocorticoid, regulates circulating fluid volume and electrolyte balance by promoting sodium and chloride retention by the distal tubule while potassium is excreted. The main active glucocorticoid cortisol generates a catabolic state that characterizes the body's response to stress by increasing blood glucose, stimulating lipolysis and generating anti-inflammatory and immunosuppressive effects.The secretion of adrenal hormones is controlled and regulated by a

*Corresponding Author's E-mail: levent.soydan@gmail.com.

negative feedback system, called the Hypothalamo-Pituitary-Adrenal Axis. Adrenal insufficiency, as identified by low levels of morning cortisol, can be primary or secondary. Primary adrenal insufficiency is caused by congenital enzymatic defects or tissue destruction from autoimmune etiology while secondary insufficiency is caused by ACTH deficiency. Primary hyperaldosteronism as identified by high aldosterone-renin ratio is a treatable disorder caused mostly by a functional adenoma. Benign functional or nonfunctional adenomas are the most common adrenal tumors while metastases to the adrenals are the most common malignant tumors. Incidentalomas which are detected incidentally may be a cause for subclinical Cushing's syndrome if they are functional. Exogenous use of excess glucocorticoids may cause Cushing Syndrome which may be lethal if not identified early and treated appropriately. Adrenal surgery can be performed laparoscopically or via an open approach. Laparoscopy can be transabdominal or posterior retroperitoneal. The surgical technique is based on the experience of the surgeon as well as on the patient and tumor characteristics.

Introduction

The adrenal hormones were fully isolated and characterized at the turn of the twentieth with adrenaline being the first isolated adrenal extract. Steroid hormones were crystallized from cortical extract by Swiss and American investigators in the 1930s, but their highly similar chemical structures made isolation of the individual compounds challenging. Kendall, Reichstein, and Hench jointly received the 1950 Nobel Prize in Physiology or Medicine for their groundbreaking work on the adrenocortical hormones. The Austrian-born endocrinologist Hans Selye first described the hypothalamic-pituitary-adrenal axis. In this chapter, we will discuss the function, regulation and common disorders of the adrenal glands.

Surgical Anatomy

The adrenal glands are located superiorly and slightly medial to the kidneys in the perirenal compartment of the retroperitoneum, which also contains the kidneys, perirenal/periadrenal fat and upper ureters. This space is bordered by Gerota's fascia anteriorly and posteriorly by the posterior renal fascia, quadratus lumborum muscle, paraspinous muscle, transversus abdominis muscle, and thoracolumbar fascia. Although there is an extensive arterial supply around the inferior, medial, and superior parts of the adrenal gland, the venous drainage is usually solitary. The left adrenal vein drains directly into the left renal vein after converging with the inferior phrenic vein. In contrast, the right adrenal vein is short, narrow, and comes off the inferior vena cava (IVC) at a near 90 degrees angle.

The adrenals are paired retroperitoneal glands that lie superiorly and anteromedially to the kidneys. They are triangular-shaped with the right adrenal gland being usually more pyramidal in shape [1]. The adrenal glands are made of an outer cortex deriving from the mesoderm and an inner medulla deriving from the neural crest. In the cortex, the zona glomerulosa produces mineralocorticoids, the zona fasciculata glucocorticoids, and the zona reticularis sex steroids or gonadocorticoids, whereas the medulla produces catecholamines, adrenaline, and noradrenaline. The adrenals are supplied by three arteries: superior (from the inferior phrenic arteries), middle (from the abdominal aorta), and inferior suprarenal arteries (from the renal arteries). The right adrenal vein ends into the inferior vena cava, while the left adrenal vein ends into the left renal vein or inferior phrenic vein. The lymphatic vessels drain to the para-aortic nodes. The innervation of adrenals comes from the splanchnic nerves arising from the aortic and renal plexuses [2].

PHYSIOLOGY

The adrenal gland is made up of the cortex and medulla. The cortex produces steroid hormones including glucocorticoids, mineralocorticoids, and adrenal androgens, and the medulla produces the catecholamines, epinephrine, and norepinephrine.

The adrenal cortexis derived from mesoderm and begins posteromedial to the urogenital ridge. The adrenal medulla is derived from neural crest. Clusters of chromaffin cells become the distinct medulla after birth [3, 4].

The adrenal cortex takes part in steroidogenesis, producing glucocorticoids, mineralocorticoids, and androgen precursors. It has 3 distinct functional and histological zones: the zona glomerulosa (outermost layer), the zona fasciculata (middle layer), and the zona reticularis (innermost layer) [5]. Each layer produces steroid hormones from one precursor element, cholesterol. Each of these specific steroid hormones are produced in different layers because of different enzymes present in each zonal layer. The zona glomerulosa produces mineralocorticoids, the zona fasciculata produces glucocorticoids, and the zona reticularis produces androgen precursors (mostly dehydroepiandrosterone [DHEA], with some androstenedione).

Following entry of the cholesterol molecule into the cell, steroidogenic acute regulatory protein (StAR) regulates cholesterol transport from the outer mitochondrial membrane to the inner mitochondrial membrane [6].In the inner mitochondrial membrane, the cholesterol can then be converted to pregnenolone via CYP11A1 (cholesterol desmolase),which acts as a catalyst in the rate-limiting step of steroid hormone production. CYP11A1 is expressed in all three layers of the adrenal cortex, and can be induced by the ACTH to promote steroidogenesis in all 3 zones. The downstream fate of pregnenolone will depend on the specific enzymes within that zone.

17 alpha-hydroxylase is not present in the glomerulosa, so pregnenolone can only be converted into progesterone by 3-beta-dehydrogenase; to 11-deoxycorticosterone by 21-hydroxylase or to corticosterone by 11-beta-hydroxylase. Aldosteron is produced by the conversion of corticosterone by aldosterone synthase, which is present only in the glomerulosa, and is regulated by angiotensin II. All of the steroids produced in the glomerulosa, namely aldosterone, corticosterone and deoxycorticosterone have mineralocorticoid activity with aldosterone, being the predominant mineralocorticoid in man.

The steroids pregnenolone and progesterone produced in the glomerulosa are converted in the fasciculata into 17-hydroxypregnenolone and 17-hydroxyprogesterone, respectively, by 17-alpha-hydroxylase. Then, 3-beta-dehydrogenase converts 17-hydroxypregnenolone into 17-hydroxyprogesterone; 21-hydroxylase converts 17-hydroxyprogesterone to

11-deoxycortisol; and 11-beta-hydroxylase converts 11-deoxycortisol to cortisol, the predominant glucocorticoid.

In the reticularis, 17-hydroxypregnenolone and 17-hydroxyprogesterone can be converted into DHEA and androstenedione by 17,20 lyase (17 alpha-hydroxylase). Although DHEA is predominantly made, some of it can be converted into androstenedione by 3ß-hydroxysteroid dehydrogenase in the reticularis.

FUNCTION

Mineralocorticoids

The mineralocorticoids, including aldosterone, corticosterone and 11-deoxycorticosterone, act on the kidney to increase sodium retention and potassium excretion. An increase in sodium reabsorption causes passive water reabsorption, leading to an increase in effective circulating volume, and therefore, increased blood pressure. To achieve this, mineralocorticoids cause increased synthesis of epithelial sodium channels (ENaC) and sodium-potassium ATPases on the principal cells of the distal nephron [7].

Mineralocorticoids also cause potassium ion secretion at the principal cells because of the gradients produced by ENaC. In hyperkalemia, aldosterone synthesis is increased to promote potassium excretion. And finally, mineralocorticoids promote hydrogen ion secretion at the intercalated cells [7].

At physiological levels,11-deoxycorticosterone and corticosterone have weaker mineralocorticoid effects compared to aldosterone but they can produce a strong mineralocorticoid effect when present in excess, as in some forms of congenital adrenal hyperplasia (CAH) or in11-beta-hydroxylase deficiency, resulting in hypertension [6].

Glucocorticoids

Cortisol is the major glucocorticoid, and increases in response to stress, which activates the HPA axis, allowing the body to function with increased stress. Upon acting on glucocorticoid receptors, cortisol increases the expression of genes that will regulate metabolism, the immune system, cardiovascular function, growth, and reproduction. Cortisol plays a role in maintaining blood pressure as it increases the sensitivity of vascular smooth muscle to vasoconstrictors like catecholamines, and inhibits the secretion of vasodilators like nitrous oxide[5].Cortisol suppresses the immune system, a feature utilized in immunosuppressive drug therapy with glucocorticoids. As for the metabolism, cortisol induces gluconeogenesis, and inhibits peripheral glucose uptake, opposing the actions of insulin, and resulting in a net increase in serum glucose. Cortisol also stimulates lipolysis and adipocyte growth causing fat deposition. Cortisol inhibits growth with associated muscle atrophy, increased bone resorption, and thinning of the skin. Although glucocorticoids can also act on mineralocorticoid receptors, the effects of aldosterone predominate in the kidney because the renal enzyme, 11-beta-hydroxysteroid dehydrogenase-2 (11-beta-HSD-2) converts cortisol to cortisone[14].The 11-beta-HSD-1 converts cortisone into cortisol. So, these enzymes constitute another set of regulation to cortisol. Licorice toxicity inhibits 11-beta-HSD-2, causing hypertension and hypokalemic alkalosis with normal aldosterone levels. Also, there can be a loss of function due to mutations in11-beta-HSD-2, resulting in hypertension with low aldosterone, as will be discussed later [9].

Androgens

DHEA constitutes most of the adrenal androgens. DHEA needs to be converted to active sex steroids in the gonads and peripheral tissue. Circulating DHEA-sulfate is the best indicator of adrenal androgen levels. Some DHEA are also converted to androstenedione. Ultimately, both of these androgens are converted to testosterone in peripheral tissues, which is converted to 5-alpha-dihydrotestosterone (DHT), the most potent androgen [6].The role of adrenal androgens in the adult male is limited as the testes are the major source of testosterone production. However, adrenal androgens do play an important role in puberty for both males and females, and are the main source of circulating testosterone in females. The rise in adrenal gland androgen synthesis is responsible for adrenarche, which precedes gonadarche [10].

Catecholamines

Adrenal catecholamines, epinephrine and norepinephrine play a role in the fight-or-flight response of the sympathetic nervous system. They act on alpha-1 receptors located on the vascular smooth, causing an increase of blood pressure. They help increase serum glucose by activating glycogenolysis and increasing glucagon secretion via beta-2 receptors, and decreasing insulin secretion via alpha-2 receptors [11].

Mechanism

Cholesterol derived from both circulating LDL and HDL forms the structural basis for the hormones made by the adrenal cortex. StaR is crucial in the delivery of cholesterol for steroidogenesis.

Clinical Significance

Adrenal pathologies can be associated with endocrine hypertension. While most causes of hypertension are primary hypertension, adrenal gland pathology can cause secondary hypertension, as in resistant hypertension caused by excess aldosterone in primary aldosteronism [12],hypertension caused by excess cortisol in Cushing syndrome [5] or hypertension caused by excess catecholamine production from a pheochromocytoma [13].On the other hand, an excess of adrenal androgen production in congenital adrenal hyperplasia (CAH) leads to ambiguous genitalia in females and isosexual precocity in males [6].

REGULATION

The Hypothalic–Pituitary–Adrenal Axis

Stress is commonly defined as a state of real or perceived threat to homeostasis. The response to stress involves activation of a complex range of endocrine, nervous, and immune system mechanisms to maintain the homeostasis in the presence of aversive stimuli (stressors).Activation of the stress response initiates a number of behavioral and physiological changes for survival. While increased awareness, improved cognition, euphoria, and enhanced analgesia are among the behavioral responses, there are a number of physiological adaptations to survival, including increased cardiovascular tone, respiratory rate and intermediate metabolism, along with inhibition of general vegetative functions, such as feeding, digestion, growth, reproduction, and immunity [17]. A wide range of tight neuronal and endocrine regulatory reactions play role in this adaptive process.

The anatomical structures that mediate the stress response are found in the central nervous system, namely the paraventricular nucleus (PVN) of the hypothalamus and the anterior lobe of the pituitary gland, as well as in the peripheral tissues (adrenal glands). This collection of structures is commonly referred to as the hypothalamic-pituitary-adrenal (HPA) axis (Figure 1). In addition to the HPA axis, several other structures play important roles in the regulation of adaptive responses to stress. These include brain stem noradrenergic neurons, sympathetic and renomedullary circuits and parasympathetic systems [18].

The hypothalamic-pituitary-adrenal (HPA) axis acts as a regulator in the production of glucocorticoids and adrenal androgens from the zona fasciculata and zona reticularis. Neurons localized in PVN produce and secrete corticotropin-releasing factor (CRF), the principle regulator of the HPA axis [19]. In response to changing circadian rhythmsor stress, CRF is released into hypophysial portal vessels that reach the anterior pituitary gland. Binding of CRF to its receptor on pituitary corticotropes induces the release of adrenocorticotropic hormone (ACTH) into the systemic circulation. CRH binds to receptors located in the adenohypophysis, leading to the production of ACTH (or corticotrophin) from pre-pro-opiomelanocortin (pre-POMC). Breakdown of POMC may also result in the production of other hormones, such as alpha-melanocyte stimulating hormone (MSH). ACTH formed in the anterior pituitary and released into the blood circulation in a pulsatile pattern that parallels the fluctuating levels of cortisol. Both ACTH and cortisol levels rise to a peak in the morning (6:00 AM to 8:00 AM) and decline throughout the day, coming to a minimum at around midnight.

Circulating ACTH induces the melanocortin type 2 receptors (MC2-R) in the zona fasciculata of the adrenal cortex to produce, mainly, the glucocorticoids. MC2-R (a G protein-coupled receptor) and MC2 receptor accessory protein (MRAP) are associated with mediating the responses to ACTH. The presence of MRAP is absolutely required for the binding and signaling of ACTH [15, 16]. Glucocorticoids regulate physiological changes through intracellular receptors in the HPA axis [20].The biological effects of glucocorticoids are usually adaptive; however, inadequate or excessive activation of the HPA axis may contribute to the development of pathologies [17]. Circulating glucocorticoids act on the hypothalamus (long loop) and the anterior pituitary (short loop), suppressing the secretion of CRH and ACTH respectively. In this way, continued rise of glucocorticoid levels is inhibited. ACTH is secreted from the anterior pituitary in a pulsatile pattern that parallels the fluctuating levels of cortisol. Both ACTH and cortisol levels rise to a peak in the morning (6:00 AM to 8:00 AM) and decline throughout the day, coming to a minimum at around midnight.

Renin-Angiotensin-Aldosterone System

The zona glomerulosa produces mineralocorticoids. While pituitary ACTH regulates adrenal glucocorticoid and androgen synthesis, mineralocorticoid synthesis is not controlled by the ACTH. Aldosterone synthesis is regulated by two factors: (1) the renin-angiotensin-aldosterone system, and (2) potassium levels. The kidney secretes renin in response to decreased renal perfusion, which is sensed by the juxtaglomerular apparatus. Renin converts angiotensinogen to angiotensin I (AT-I), which is then converted to angiotensin II (AT-II) via angiotensin-converting enzyme in the lung. AT-II stimulates aldosterone synthesis in the zona glomerulosa by activating aldosterone synthase [21].

Adrenal Medulla

The secretion of epinephrine and norepinephrine from the adrenal medulla is controlled and regulated by the sympathetic nervous system [22].

The CRF Family of Peptides

In the brain, CRF is concentrated in the medial parvocellular subdivision of the PVN, and is also localized in the olfactory bulb, bed nucleus of the stria terminalis, medial preoptic area, lateral hypothalamus, centralnucleus of the amygdala, Barington's nucleus, dorsal motor complex and inferior olive. In the periphery, CRF has been detected in the adrenal gland, testis, placenta, gastrointestinal tract, thymus, and skin [23].

The neuroendocrine properties of CRF are mediated through CRFRl in the anterior pituitary. Binding of CRF to the type 1 receptor results in the stimulation of adenylate cyclase, and a subsequent activation of cAMP pathway events that culminate with the release of ACTH from pituitary corticotropes [24].The neuroendocrine effects of CRF are modulated by CRF binding proteins that are found at high levels in the systemic circulation and in the pituitary gland [25].

Vasopressin

Vasopressin (AVP) is a nanopeptide that is highly expressed in the PVN, supraoptic, and suprachiasmatic nuclei of the hypothalamus [17].It potentiates the effects of CRF on ACTH release from the anterior pituitary [26]. The synergistic effects of AVP on ACTH release are mediated through the vasopressin V_{1b}receptor on pituitary corticotropes [27].AVP plays an important role in the stress response by maintaining ACTH responsiveness to novel stressors during periods of chronic stress.

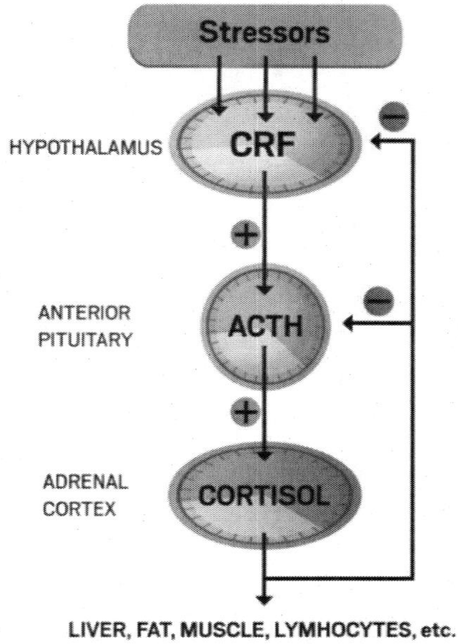

Figure 1. Schematic representation of the hypothalamic-pituitary-adrenal (HPA) axis. Hypophysiotropic neurons in the paraventricular nucleus of the hypothalamus produce corticotropin-releasing factor (CRF) and vasopressin. In response to stress, CRF is released into hypophysial portal vessels that access the anterior pituitary gland. Binding of CRF to the CRF type 1 receptor on pituitary corticotropes induces the release of adrenocorticotropic hormone (ACTH) into the systemic circulation. Circulating ACTH binds to the melanocortin type 2 receptor (MC2-R) in the adrenal cortex where it stimulates glucocorticoid synthesis and secretion into the systemic circulation. Glucocorticoids regulate physiological events and inhibit further HPA axis activation through intracellular receptors that are widely distributed throughout peripheral tissues.

Adrenocorticotropic Hormone

Pro-opiomelanocortin (POMC) is a prohormone abundant in the pituitary and the hypothalamus. POMC is processed into a number of bioactive peptides including ACTH, β-endorphin, β-lipotropic hormone, and the melanocortins [28].In response to CRF, ACTH is released from pituitary corticotropes into the systemic circulation, where it binds to its specific receptor in the adrenal cortex. ACTH binds to the melanocortin type 2 receptor (MC2-R) in parenchymal cells of the adrenocortical zona fasciculata. Activation of the MC2-R induces stimulation of cAMP pathway events that induce steroidogenesis and the secretion of glucocorticoids, mineral corticoids, and androgenic steroids [29].Specifically, ACTH promotes the conversion of cholesterol into 5-5 pregnenolone during the initial step of glucocorticoid biosynthesis [28].

Endocrine Regulation of the HPA Axis

Activation of the HPA axis is a tightly controlled process involving a series of neuronal and endocrine systems. Glucocorticoids are key elements in regulating the magnitude and duration of HPA axis activation [17].Following exposure to stress, elevated levels of circulating glucocorticoids inhibit HPA activity at the level of the hypothalamus and pituitary. The HPA axis has also an intrinsic regulation that is independent of glucocorticoids.

Glucocorticoid Negative Feedback

The HPA axis is controlled by feedback inhibition from circulating glucocorticoids [17]. Glucocorticoids act on the HPA axis through at least two distinct paths of negative feedback. It is well known that glucocorticoids inhibit activation of the HPA axis through a delayed feedback system that is sensitive to glucocorticoid levels, and involves genomic alterations. However, a fast nongenomic feedback system appears to play an additional role that is also responsive the level of glucocorticoids. The exact mechanism of this second rapid feedback system has not been clarified yet [20].

The delayed feedback system acts via transcriptional alterations, and is regulated by glucocorticoid receptors (GR), localized in a number of stress-responsive brain regions [17]. Glucocorticoids have a low nanomolar affinity for the GR, and extensively occupy GRs during periods of elevated glucocorticoid secretion that occur following stress [17]. Mineralocorticoid receptors (MRs) have a subnanomolar affinity for glucocorticoids, a restricted expression pattern in the brain, and bind glucocorticoids during periods of basal secretion [30].Therefore, it appears that MRs regulate basal HPA tone, while GRs mediate glucocorticoid negative feedback, following stress [17].

PVN is an important site for glucocorticoid feedback inhibition of the HPA axis. The hippocampus appears to be a second site for the regulation of HPA axis via a glucocorticoid negative feedback. The hippocampus contains a high concentration of both GR and MR, and exposure to glucocorticoids reduces basal and stress induced glucocorticoid release [31].

Neuronal Regulation of the HPA Axis

Most afferent inputs to the PVN originate from four distinct regions in the brain: brainstem neurons, lamina terminalis, extra-PVN hypothalamic nuclei, and forebrain limbic structures [32]. These cell groups relay information about a wide range of sensory modalities to affect CRF expression and release from hypophysiotropic neurons of the PVN.

Brain Stem Neurons

Brain stem catecholaminergic centers play an important role in the regulation of the HPA axis. Afferent sensory information from cranial nerves that innervate large areas of thoracic and abdominal viscera is transmitted by neurons of the nucleus of the solitary tract (NTS) to the PVN. The NTS also receives projections from limbic structures that regulate behavioral responses to stress, including the medial prefrontal cortex and the central nucleus of the amygdala [17]. Catecholaminergic input excites the HPA axis, and causes CRF expression and protein release through an α-1 adrenergic receptor-dependent mechanism [33].

Nonaminergic NTS neurons, Glucagon-like peptide 1 containing neurons,neuropeptides somatostatin, substance P, and enkephalin all innervate the PVN and contribute to HPA axis regulation [34].

The Lamina Terminals

Cell groups of the lamina terminalis relay information concerning the osmotic composition of blood to the PVN [35]. The PVN receives rich innervation from the subfornical organ, which sends angiotensinergic neurons to the PVN, and induce CRF secretion and biosynthesis [36].This afferent pathway may be a link between HPA and neurohypophysial activation [37].

Hypothalamus

The medial parvocellular subdivision of the PVN receives afferent projections from y-aminobutyric acid GABAergic neurons of the hypothalamus [17]. GABA plays a prominent role in hypothalamic stress integration. GABAergic neurons in the dorsomedial hypothalamic nucleus and preoptic area (POA) project to the medial parvocellular division of the PVN, and are activated following exposure to stressors [38]. The POA is a potential site of integration between gonadal steroids and the HPA axis. So, neurons of the POA are activated by gonadal steroids, and express high levels of androgen, estrogen and progesterone receptors [39].

Hypothalamic centers involved in the regulation of energy homeostasis directly innervate PVN neurons. Neurons in the arcuate nucleus are sensitive to circulating levels of glucose, insulin and leptin. Arcuate neuropeptides have significant effects on HPA axis activity. The HPA axis is activated in response to positive and negative states of energy balance. Limbic structures of the forebrain also contribute to the regulation of the HPA axis. Neuronal populations in the hippocampus, prefrontal cortex and amygdala are related to memory formation and emotional responses, and may serve as a link between the stress system and neuropsychiatric disorders [40].The hippocampus, prefrontal cortex and amygdala have significant effects on glucocorticoid release and behavioral responses to stress [41].However, these limbic structures are thought to regulate HPA axis activity through intermediary neurons in hypothalamus and brain stem [42].

The hippocampus plays an important role in the terminating HPA axis responses to stress as evidenced by elevated basal levels of circulating glucocorticoids, prolonged ACTH and corticosterone release, in response to stress in patients with hippocampal lesions [17]. The prefrontal cortex also regulates HPA responses to stress. In acute and chronic stress states, neurons of the medial prefrontal cortex are activated, and release catecholamines [38]. The prefrontal cortex may also inhibit HPA axis through glucocorticoid feedback inhibition. In contrast to the hippocampus and the prefrontal cortex, the amygdala is thought to activate the HPA axis. Stimulation of amygdalar neurons promotes synthesis and release of glucocorticoids into the systemic circulation [43].

Activation of brain stem noradrenergic neurons and sympathetic and renomedullary circuits further contribute to the body's response to stressful stimuli. Similar to the HPA axis, stress-evoked activation of the locus coeruleus induces norepinephrine and subsequent ACTH release along with anxiogenic-like behaviors and suppression of immune functions [17].

Disorders

Tumors of the Adrenal Gland with Imaging Features

Adrenal glands are site to various pathological processes, including hyperplasia, hemorrhage, benign and malignant tumors. Suspicion of a hyperfunctioning adrenal lesion may arise when patients present with respective symptoms, leading to examination by imaging methods. Conversely, non-functioning adrenal lesions may be detected incidentally on imaging when patients are examined to investigate another potential pathology. The increased application of adrenal imaging methods, including ultrasound (US), Computed Tomography (CT) and Magnetic Resonance (MR) has led to an increased detection of these incidental lesions.

Incidental adrenal masses are common, occurring in about 3-7% of adults, with the majority of these lesions being benign non-functioning adenomas [44]. Imaging helps in the differentiation between benign and malignant adrenal lesions because this affects the clinical management of patients.

Both CT and MR have pivotal roles in adrenal imaging. CT represents the first-level imaging modality for the evaluation of adrenal lesions, thanks to its ability to deliver a quick examination with high spatial resolution [45]. MR still remains a second-level modality, with advantages including multiparametricity, multiplanarity, higher contrast resolution in comparison with CT, and the added value of chemical shift imaging (CSI) [46].

US has a limited part in the assessment of adrenals due to its low accuracy in the detection and characterization of small adrenal neoplasms, compared to CT and MR. Still, US can be used to differentiate a cystic from a solid mass, and in neonatal patients where the adrenals are bigger compared to the kidneys, US may still have a role in imaging.

In clinically functioning adrenal lesions, nuclear medicine techniques such as scintigraphy with 131/123I-meta-iodo-benzyl-guanidine (MIBG) and Octreotide can be used. Moreover, positron emission tomography (PET) has also shown to be helpful for the evaluation of non-hyperfunctioning adrenal masses with high accuracy in the characterization of malignant lesions [47].

Finally, adrenal imaging is also important preoperatively to determine the position of the tumor within the gland, and the relationship of the adrenal/tumor to the renal hilum, kidney, and major vasculature.

Adenoma

Adenoma is the most common benign adrenal tumor. It arises from the cortex and has no malignant transformation. It consists of clear cells with abundant intracytoplasmatic fat. Typically, the remaining portion of the adrenal gland and the contralateral adrenal appear atrophic. Large adenomas may show cystic components, calcifications, and hemorrhagic areas. Incidence of adenomas increases with age. Most are non-functioning, and therefore generally asymptomatic, and are detected incidentally (incidentaloma) [48]. Hyperfunctioning adrenal adenomas present with symptoms and signs related to excess hormone secretion, thereby leading to Cushing's syndrome (hyperproduction of cortisol) or Conn's syndrome (hyperproduction of aldosterone), while they rarely lead to an adrenal-genital syndrome [49].

The typical adenoma measures less than 3cm, making its detection challenging through US, where it appears as a homogeneous and hypoechoic solid lesion with well-defined margins, hypovascularization on

Color Doppler examination, and hypoenhancing on contrast-enhanced US (CEUS) [49]. At unenhanced CT, adenomas are usually well-demarcated round or oval lesions, with homogeneous and relatively low attenuation values (lower than 10 Hounsfield Units [HU]), due to high fat content [50]. However, unenhanced CT alone is not always diagnostic, since 15–30% of adenomas are lipid-poor with higher attenuation values. In these cases, intravenous contrast administration is required to differentiate adenomas from non-adenomas. The evaluation of the enhancement pattern of adrenal lesions needs a further late phase after the acquisition of the venous phase. A CT protocol with a 15-min post-contrast delay has been reported as having the highest diagnostic accuracy [49].

Absolute percentage washout (APW) is calculated using the following formula:

(enhanced HU−15-min delayed HU) / (enhanced HU−unenhanced HU) x100%

Relative percentage washout (RPW) is used when unenhanced CT value is not available, and the enhanced values are compared to 15-min delayed scans, by using the following formula:

(enhanced HU−15-min delayed HU) / (enhanced HU) x 100%

If the APW is >60% or RPW is >40% after 15-min from contrast administration, this is indicative of adenoma, with sensitivity and specificity of 88% and 96% at the APW and sensitivity and specificity of 83% and 93% at the RPW, respectively [45]. This method enables to differentiate adenomas that enhance quickly and show rapid washout, from non-adenomas such as metastases, which instead demonstrate strong enhancement but prolonged washout. Another useful imaging feature is the size and dimensional growth of the lesion. That is; adrenal lesions greater than 4 cm have the potential to be malignant and adenomas grow slower than malignant lesions [51].

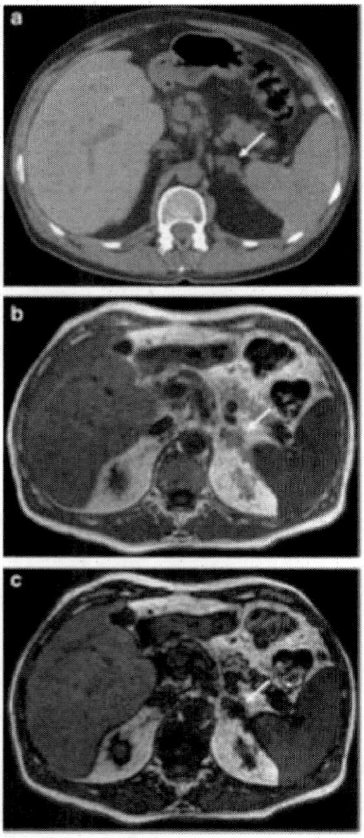

Figure 2. Left adrenal adenoma. a) Unenhanced CT shows lesion with attenuation <10HU. b) Axial in-phase and c) Out-phase T1 sequences with loss of signal intensity suggesting presence of intralesional fat. Ref: [49].

MR has a similar diagnostic accuracy to CT, allowing characterizing adenomas, regardless of their CT enhancement (Figure 2). On T2-weighted MR images, adrenal adenomas are homogeneous, and present intermediate-low signal intensity, compared to skeletal muscle or liver; intra-lesional hemorrhage can occur in large adenomas, resulting in hyperintense areas on T1-weighted images [49]. An important component of adrenal MR protocol is chemical shift imaging which enables to detect intra-lesional fat in adenomas resulting in a loss of signal intensity in the opposed phased images (Figure 2) [46].

Most adrenal adenomas demonstrate a loss of signal intensity on out-of-phase images, and a decrease in signal intensity of more than 20% is considered diagnostic of adenoma. Contrast-enhanced CT (CECT) remains the gold standard technique, especially in the evaluation of lipid-poor adenomas. Dual energy CT allows an accurate characterization of lipid-rich adenoma, evaluating that a decrease in attenuation of an adrenal lesion between 140 and 80 kVp is a highly specific sign of adenoma; but because of an overlap of attenuation values of metastatic lesions at 80 kVp the sensitivity of this modality is still low [52].A newer method called histogram analysis on unenhanced CT has been reported to have high accuracy and specificity in identifying adenomas [53].

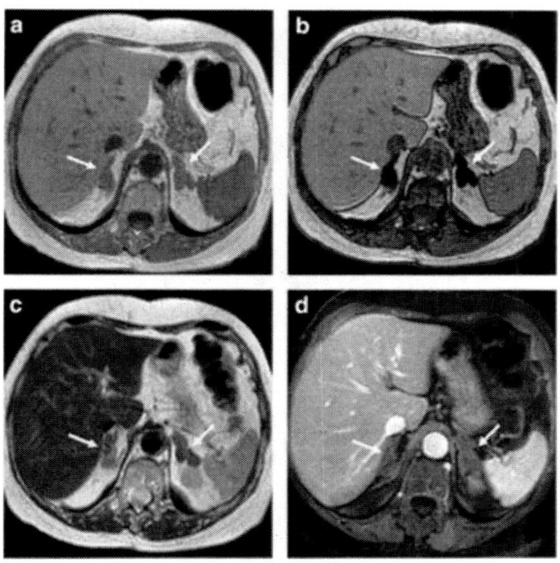

Figure 3. Bilateral adrenal hyperplasia. Nodular enlargement of both adrenals with loss of signal from a) In-phase to b) out-phase T1 sequences. c) T2 weighted and d) Postcontrast T1 weighted images with no prominent enhancement of adrenal glands. Ref: [49].

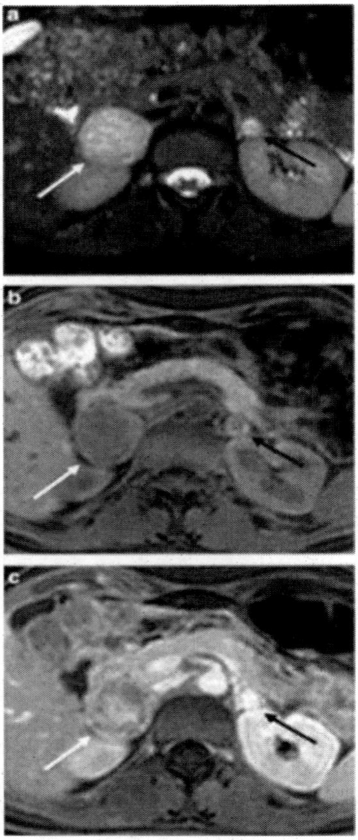

Figure 4. Bilateral adrenal pheochromocytomas in MEN-type 2. a) T2 sequence with hyperintense adrenal lesions. b) Pre and c) Postcontrast T1 sequences show enhancement of both adrenal lesions. Ref: [49].

Hyperplasia

Hyperplasia refers to nonmalignant diffuse or nodular enlargement of the adrenal gland, which is an uncommon cause of ACTH-independent Cushing's syndrome or Conn's syndrome. Adrenal hyperplasia can be congenital or acquired, and is classified according to morphology in diffuse or nodular adrenal hyperplasia. Primary pigmented nodular adrenal disease causes ACTH-independent Cushing's syndrome, and is a benign condition, generally characterized by mild symptoms related to hypercortisolism. In patients with PPNAD, imaging allows to identify multiple small nodules in normal-sized or enlarged adrenal glands [49].

At CT, diffuse hyperplasia is characterized by the nodular enlargement of both adrenals, presenting smooth margins, a homogeneous structure and often some nodules of variable size, usually smaller than 5–10 mm, but even up to 2 cm. A large nodule is rarely detected and it differs from the adenoma because the former lies within enlarged glands, while the latter appears within an atrophic adrenal gland, or associated with atrophy of the contralateral gland. Hyperplasia contains variably sized groups of lipid-rich cells, thereby showing a significant overlap with adenoma in terms of lesion attenuation [49].

On MR, hyperplasia shows signal intensity similar to that of the normal gland but appears as homogeneous or nodular enlarged gland. This appearance helps in the differentiation from other nodular pathologies, which are generally hyperintense on T2-weighted images (Figure 3) [49].

Myelolipoma

Adrenal lipomatous tumors are neoplasms with significant amounts of adipose tissue. Myelolipoma is the most common among them. It is a benign tumor, usually unilateral, small, and often incidentally discovered. It consists of mature fat and hematopoietic cells from myeloid, erythroid and megakaryocytic lines. The fat content is variable. Calcifications, partial replacement by hemorrhage or fibrosis may rarely be seen. Large lesions tend to become symptomatic due to pressure effects and intra-lesional hemorrhage or infarctions.

At US, fat-predominant lesions appear hyperechoic, while myelolipomas mainly composed of myeloid elements appear hypoechoic. Frequently, the lesion has mixed hyperechoic and hypoechoic areas due to varying amount of fat and myeloid elements [54].

At CT, myelolipoma appears as a round mass with well-defined borders. The density varies depending on the proportion of fat and myeloid components. Internal inhomogeneity is related to intra-lesional septa, necrosis, hemorrhage or calcifications. Thus, myelolipoma goes from totally fat lesions with thin circles of parenchymatous tissue to clearly parenchymatous forms with small areas of fat. At CT, myelolipoma is easily diagnosed with fat attenuation values < -30 HU. Slight postcontrast enhancement is seen due to poor vascularization [54].

On MR, the fat macroscopic components are hyperintense on T1- and T2-weighted images, while the hematopoietic parts are hypointense on T1- and moderately hyperintense on T2-weighted images. The diagnosis is verified with signal drop of the hyperintensity on T1-weighted images upon fat suppression [54]. Similar to renal angiomyolipomas, the presence of the India ink artifact on CSI at the myelolipoma-adrenal interface or within an adrenal mass on opposed-phase images indicates a myelolipoma [49]. Fat-suppressed images show greater loss of signal intensity than CSI sequences, as the presence of macroscopic adipose tissue is typical of myelolipoma (Figure 5). On contrast-enhanced MR, myelolipoma may have enhancement of the myeloid component. Based on MR characteristics, three different types of myelolipoma are described. The first is mostly composed of fat and homogeneous, and hyperintense on T1-weighted images. The second consisted of similar content of fat and myeloid components with a heterogeneous appearance. The third type is mainly composed of myeloid tissue with enhancement after contrast injection [49].

Pheochromocytoma

Pheochromocytoma arises from the chromaffin cells of the adrenal medulla, and typically produces both norepinephrine and epinephrine [49]. Extra-adrenal pheochromocytomas are called paragangliomas, and arise from the sympathetic ganglia at the level of the mediastinum, abdomen and pelvis. Adrenal pheochromocytoma is mostly benign, with 10% being malignant [49]. Malignant pheochromocytomas are recognized for local infiltration or metastases, usually involving the bone, liver, lymph nodes, lungs and brain. Clinical symptoms are associated with catecholamine excess. This tumor is generally sporadic but occasionally seen with hereditary syndromes, including multiple endocrine neoplasia (MEN)-2A, MEN-2B (50%), von Hippel-Lindau (10-20%), and Neurofibromatosis-1 (3%). In these cases, the adrenal lesions are usually bilateral or in form of paragangliomas. Pheochomocytomas have also been associated with other very rare genetic syndromes, including MEN-1, Carney Complex, Beckwith-Wiedeman, Li-Fraumeni syndrome and familial adenomatous polyposis [55]. Pheochromocytomas range from 1.2 to 15 cm in size [49]. If pheochromocytoma is suspected, plasma or urine metanephrines should be assessed.

Imaging of pheochromocytomas is often challenging due to its complex and variable appearance due to necrosis, fibrosis, cystic and fatty degeneration and calcification; and thus, they can mimicother lesions [49].

At US, pheochromocytomas are heterogeneous and well-encapsulated, with hypervascularization at color Doppler and an early arterial pattern of enhancement at CEUS [56].

At CT, they can show solid, cystic, calcific, and/or necrotic components. Smaller tumors tend to display a more uniform attenuation, with a density of 40–50 UH [56]. After contrast administration, pheochromocytomas enhance avidly with some of them showing higher enhancement on the portal venous phase, and others, on the arterial phase. Nevertheless, their APW and RPW are similar to those of adenomas [56]. Therefore, pheochromocytomas often cannot be reliably differentiated from adenomas using CT washout protocols. Whenlesionsare quite large (> 6 cm), intra-lesional hemorrhage, necrosis or calcifications can be observed, determining the inhomogenous contrast enhancement.

MR has high sensitivity for the diagnosis of pheochromocytomas (about 98%) [56]. Pheochromocytoma is slightly hypointense on T1-weighted, and hyperintense on T2-weighted images (Figure 4) [49]. No signal loss is seen on opposed-phase images as in the case of a typical adenoma. In cases with areas of fatty degeneration, there may be a slight signal drop on CSI [46].

Targeted PET imaging with 68Ga-DOTA-peptides enables to detect expression of somatostatin receptors by pheochromocytoma [49].18F-FDOPA PET/CT can show uptake and storage of catecholamines in pheochromocytomas and enables potential evaluation of the relationship between tumor secretion and its biochemical phenotype [57].

Uncommon Benign Adrenal Lesions

Cyst

Adrenal cysts are classified as pseudocysts (resulting from previous hemorrhage), endothelial cysts (with a thin endothelial wall and lactescent liquid, deriving from lymphangiectasia or arteriovenous malformations), epithelial cysts (with thin epithelial wall and serous liquid content), and parasitic cysts (hydatid disease). These cysts can range in size from 1 to 20cm [49]. At US, endothelial and epithelial cysts appear as well-circumscribed hypoechoic or anechoic lesions with thin walls, while pseudocysts may have thicker walls. The scattered echogenicity, the presence of debris, or fluid-fluid levels suggest previous hemorrhage into a pseudocyst [49].

On CT, adrenal cysts appear as well-demarcated, non-enhancing, hypodense lesion with water attenuation (< 20 HU) and thin walls.

On MR, cysts are usually hyperintense on T2-weighted images (Figure 4). Pseudocysts may contain septations, blood products, soft-tissue components and calcifications [49].

Lipoma

Adrenal lipomas are of mesenchymal origin, containing mature fatty tissue, and surrounded by a fibrous capsule. These are well-demarcated lesions, composed of lobules of fat tissue. On CT, in contrast to myelolipomas, they show no or minimal soft-tissue attenuation, and can contain focal areas of intra-lesional calcifications due to degenerative changes [49].

Hemangioma

Hemangioma is an incidental adrenal lesion, generally discovered by CT or MR, especially in women between 40 and 70 years of age. Regarding the histologic types, the most common are capillary and cavernous hemangiomas [49]. On US, hemangioma has no specific characteristics, appearing as a mass with variable size and echotexture. On CT, small hemangiomas can be homogeneous, whereas larger lesions present calcifications, which can be either phleboliths or dystrophic calcifications due to previous hemorrhages. On CECT, hemangioma shows heterogeneous and mainly peripheral enhancement, with or without central filling on delayed phases (Figure 6). At MR, hemangioma is hypointense on T1-weighted with a remarkable hyperintensity on T2-weighted images (lightbulb sign). Hypointense foci can be encountered on T1- and T2-weighted images related to intra-lesional calcifications. Also on contrast-enhanced MR, hemangioma usually displays peripheral nodular enhancement [49].

Lymphangioma

Lymphangiomas are incidentally discovered benign adrenal lesions. On CT, lymphangioma appears as a well-encapsulated hypodense lesion (8–20 HU) with an average size of 3 cm with intra-lesional septations and with post-contrast enhancement. At MR, there are no specific imaging features [49].

Schwannoma

Schwannoma is usually a benign and asymptomatic tumor, arising from the sheath of the nerves. CT and MR features are non-specific. Larger lesions usually present degenerative changes, including hemorrhagic components, calcifications and cystic areas with respective imaging features.

Ganglioneuroma

Ganglioneuroma is a benign tumor, arising from the sympathetic nerves or within the adrenals. Adrenal medulla is a less frequent location compared to the mediastinum or the retroperitoneum. Usually, it is a small round mass (2–3cm) with well-defined smooth margins and an inhomogeneous appearance due to mixoid components. On CT, it may display calcifications, necrosis, and hemorrhagic areas [49]. It remains hypoattenuating on early post-contrast phases, while becoming hyperattenuating on delayed phases due to persistent enhancement.

On MR, ganglioneuroma is hypointense on T1-weighted, and hyperintense on T2-weighted images, with gradual and progressive enhancement on post-contrast sequences [49].

Adenomatoid Tumor

Adenomatoid tumor is of an asymptomatic lesion of mesothelial origin. On CECT, this tumor appears hypodense with heterogeneous contrast enhancement. MR findings are non-specific [49].

Oncocytoma

Oncocytoma is an epithelial tumor. It involves mostly the left adrenal, attaining larger sizes with a mean size of about 9cm. This neoplasm is generally benign and non-functioning. According to the Lin-Weiss-Bisceglia criteria, adrenal oncocytomas can be benign, borderline malignant potential and malignant lesions. They rarely metastasize. On CT and MR scans, the lesion shows fibrous encapsulation [49]. Differentiation of oncocytoma from cortical carcinoma is difficult [56].

Other Conditions Affecting the Adrenal Glands

Adrenal Infection

Tuberculosis is one the most frequent adrenal infections, still being the primary cause of primary adrenal insufficiency in developing countries. Tuberculosis affects usually both adrenal glands, leading to symptoms of adrenal insufficiency, including weakness, nausea, anorexia, weight loss, abdominal pain, and hypotension. CT and MR show different imaging findings depending on stage. At first, a mass-like enlargement with preserved contour is commonly detected. Unenhanced CT shows central low attenuation, while post-contrast CT and MR images show peripheral enhancement due to central caseous necrosis [49]. Ultimately, a decrease in size of adrenal glands ensues often with diffuse, localized or punctuated calcifications.

Atrophic adrenal glands with calcifications are therefore considered highly suspicious for chronic tuberculosis. During antituberculosis therapy, the caseous necrosis can be replaced by fibrous tissue, thereby leading to a more homogeneous enhancement or central calcific deposits [58]. Another adrenal infection, mimicking tuberculosis, is histoplasmosis, although neoplastic conditions, such as metastases or lymphoma may show similar imaging features. Therefore, histologic evaluation of adrenal tissue after biopsy is generally needed to reach a correct diagnosis.

Adrenal Hemorrhage

Adrenal hemorrhage can be caused by trauma, anticoagulant therapy, complicated pregnancy, sepsis or stress, such as surgery [59]. Adrenal hemorrhage may also be found in adenoma, myelolipoma, pheochromocytoma, metastasis and cortical carcinoma. Trauma is the most common cause and it is usually unilateral [49]. Bilateral hemorrhage occurs in 20% of cases, and adrenal insufficiency secondary to hemorrhage is extremely rare [59].

US represents the first-level imaging modality in children. Acute hemorrhage appears as a mass with a diameter of 3–4cm with a mixed echostructure, predominantly hyperechogenic due to blood clots within the hematoma. Later, the mass progressively undergoes liquification, and becomes hypo-anechoic due to the lysis of the clots. At Color Doppler, adrenal hemorrhage shows no vascularization [59].

On CT, acute hemorrhage is characterized by high attenuation values in post-traumatic cases, associated with hemorrhagic suffusion of periadrenal fat and retroperitoneal bleeding (Figure 3). A chronic hematoma appears as a mass with a hypoattenuating center, with or without calcifications, which is also termed as "adrenal pseudocyst." Hematomas usually decrease in size and may spontaneously disappear. Calcifications may develop in later stages [59].

On MR, signal intensity of adrenal hemorrhage depends on its stage. In the acute stage (first 7 days), the hematoma appears isointense or slightly hypointense on T1-weighted and hypointense on T2-weighted images due to the presence of deoxyhemoglobin. In the subacute phase (1 week to 7 weeks), the hemorrhage appears hyperintense on both T1- and T2-weighted images due to the paramagnetic effect of the methemoglobin. In the chronic stage (more than 7 weeks), a hypointense rim on T1- and T2-weighted images due to hemosiderin deposition and fibrosis is detectable [59].

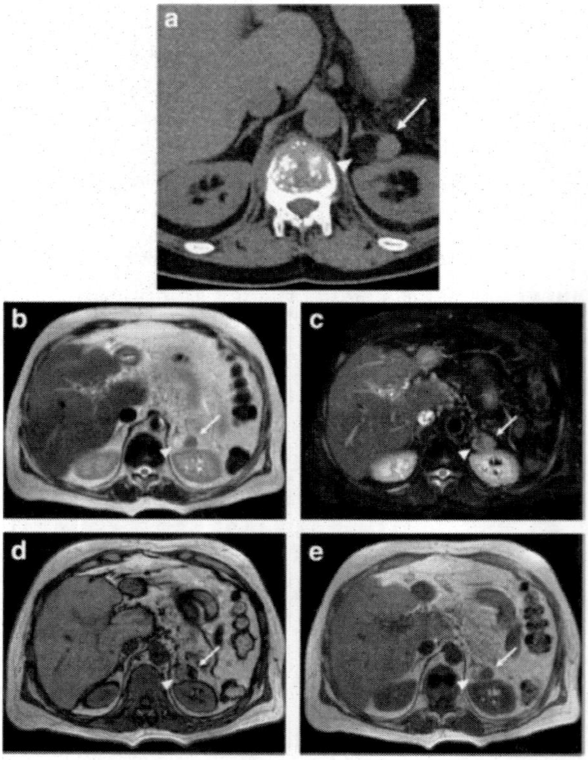

Figure 5.Left adrenal myelolipoma. (a) Unenhanced CT showsa left adrenal mass with macroscopic fat (arrowhead) and a soft-tissue myeloid component (arrow). (b) Axial T2-weighted fast spin echo. (c) T2-weighted fat-saturated spin echo. (d) T1-weightedout-of-phase and (e) in-phasegradient recalled echo images. Figure c) shows the signal drop of macroscopic fat in fatsuppressed T2-weigthed images (arrowhead) and Figure d) shows loss of signal on out-of-phase imaging of the myeloid element (arrow). Ref: [49].

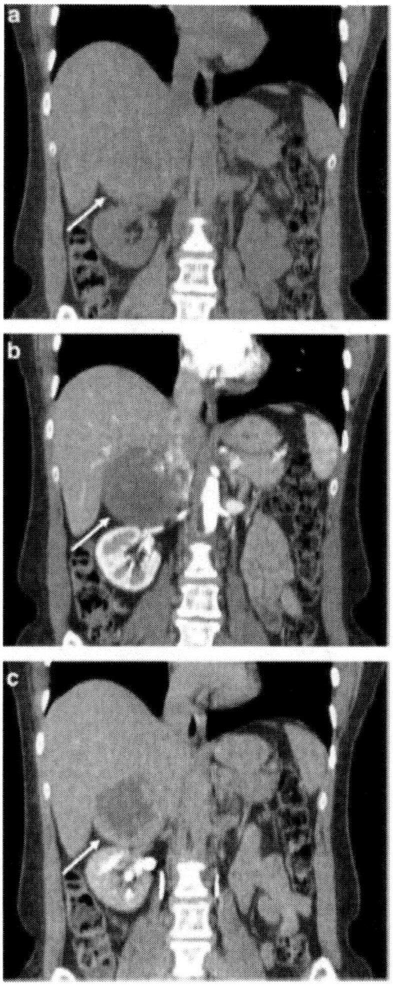

Figure 6. Right adrenal hemangioma. Coronal reformatted a) non-contrast, b) early and c) late postcontrast CTshow a well-encapsulatedright adrenal lesion (arrow) showing peripheral contrast enhancement with progressive centripetal filling and characteristic of a hemangioma. Ref: [49].

Malignant Adrenal Tumors

Metastases

Metastases are the most frequent malignant adrenal lesions. By far the most common primary tumor metastasizing to the adrenal glands is the broncogenic carcinoma, followed by breast, colon, melanoma, kidney and hepatocellular carcinoma [49]. Bilateral metastases are more common than unilateral metastases [49]. Metastases do not usually cause symptoms, but in some cases, extensive involvement of both glands can lead to adrenal insufficiency. CT is the method of choice in oncologic patients, while US is used predominantly in pediatric patients.MR is a second-instance method, useful only for further characterization of adrenal lesions. 18F-FDG-PET/CT can be helpful to differentiate fat poor adenoma from small metastasis [60].

At CT, adrenal metastases present as focal masses with strong and prolonged enhancement on the portal venous phase, usually measuring more than 120 HU, but the washout is slower than adenomas (Figure 6) [49].

At MR, imaging features depend on the type of primary tumor, but generally appear hypointense on T1-weighted and moderately hyperintense on T2-weighted images. Metastases from melanoma may be hyperintense on T1-weighted images. Moreover, if adrenal metastases contain hemorrhagic intra-lesional components, hypointense areas on T2-weighted images with no postcontrast enhancement may be seen. Adrenal metastases do not show signal loss on out-of-phase images in contrast to adenomas [49]. However, differentiation of metastasis from primary carcinoma is very challenging, with carcinoma generally showing higher local invasiveness [61].

As a functional imaging modality, which provides glucose metabolic information on malignant tumors, 18F-FDG-PET/CT has shown encouraging results for the detection of adrenal metastases. Diagnostic performance of 18F-FDG-PET/CT has been reported to be promising in the differentiation of adrenal metastases from benign masses (Figure 7) [62]. Given the high reported specifity, especially in cases with unenhanced attenuation of >10 HU at CT imaging and a SUV max ratio of >2.5 in PET, the use of 18F-FDG-PET/CT could be considered as a second-stage imaging study for evaluation of indeterminate adrenal lesions [49].

Neuroblastoma

Neuroblastoma ranks second in childhood tumors after Wilms tumor. It is very rare in adults. This lesion usually presents calcification, necrosis, and intra-lesional hemorrhage. Generally, it is totally asymptomatic; symptoms only arise when it invades or compresses adjacent structures, metastasizes, or causes paraneoplastic clinical findings [49].

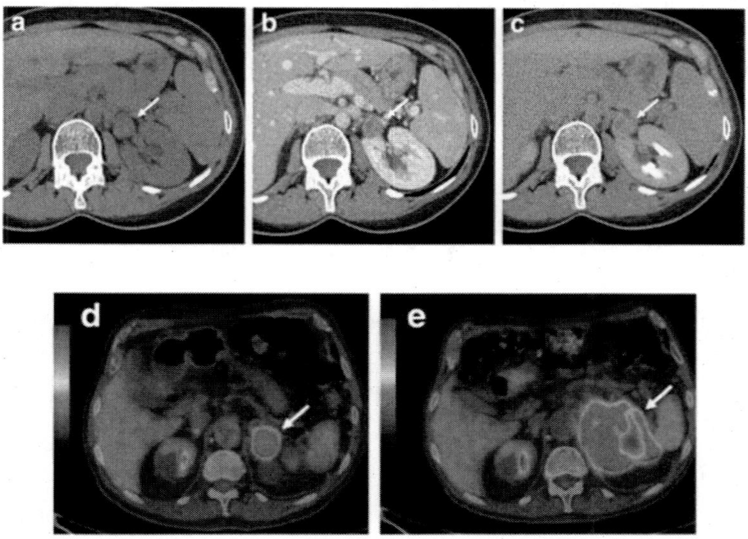

Figure 7. Left adrenal metastasis. a) Unenhanced CT. b) Postcontrast portal phase CT and c) late phase images showing 15% absolute washout in lesion. d) FDG-PET/CT images with high metabolic activity on the lesion. e) postchemotherapy PET image showing lesion with central necrosis. Ref: [49].

US is the first imaging modality for this lesion in pediatric patients. Neuroblastoma presents as a large lesion with inhomogeneous echotexture, intra-lesional vascularity at color Doppler, and sometimes with calcifications [63]. On CT, it is a lobulated mass, with amorphous or mottled calcifications, usually without capsule and shows mild postcontrast enhancement. Intra-lesional calcifications are detected in 80–90% of cases, and when present, they constitute a clue to differentiate it from Wilms tumor [63].

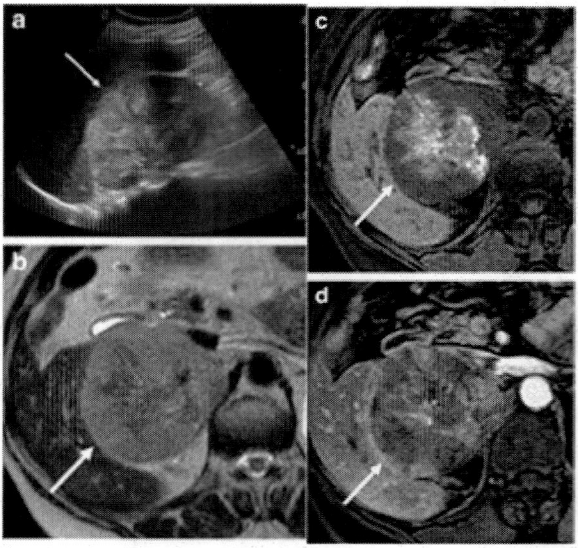

Figure 8. Right adrenal cortical carcinoma. a) Sonography shows heterogeneous adrenal mass. b)T2 weighted image. c) Precontrast T1 image shows high signal areas suggesting intralesional hemorrhage. d) No prominent enhancement in postcontrast T1 image. Ref: [49].

MR has been reported to be more accurate than CT in the characterization. Neuroblastoma usually shows a variable appearance, hypointense on T1-weighted and hyperintense on T2-weighted images, with heterogeneous postcontrast enhancement [63].

Detection of neuroblastoma by MIBG scintigraphy has been reported to be of equal sensitivity to that for pheochromocytoma [49].

Rare Malignant Adrenal Tumors

Lymphoma

Secondary lymphomatous adrenal involvement is seen more frequent than the primary lymphoma [49]. In 50% of cases, a bilateral adrenal involvement with associated retroperitoneal lymphadenopathy is seen [64]. On US, lymphoma appears as hypoechoic with a homogenous or heterogeneous appearance. On CT, primary adrenal lymphoma appears as a single hypodense mass, without intra-lesional calcifications, with minimal post contrast enhancement [49]. In secondary adrenal lymphoma, the adrenals appear homogenously enlarged but maintain normal morphology. Postcontrast secondary lymphomas show slight contrast enhancement and slow washout [64]. At MR, adrenal lymphoma is hypo/isointense on T1-weighted and slightly hyperintense on T2-weighted images [64]. On DWI, lymphomatous lesions always show a restricted pattern of diffusion due to their hypercellularity butthis is not specific for adrenal lymphoma [49].

Cortical Carcinoma

Cortical carcinoma has a bimodal peak of incidence in childhood and middle age. They may be functioning especially in females. There may be an association with endocrine syndromes, including Li-Fraumeni syndrome, Beckwith-Wiedemann syndrome, Carney complex, congenital adrenal hyperplasia and MEN-1 [49]. Non-functioning lesions remain asymptomatic unless they cause compression and dislocation of adjacent structures.

At US, they are detected when they are larger than 6 cm in size, where they appear heterogeneous due to necrosis or hemorrhage. Smaller lesions may show more homogeneous echotexture. Echogenic foci due to calcifications may be observed. At Color Doppler, this lesion appears as a hypervascular mass, which may demonstrate an afferent blood vessel. CEUS reveals a hypervascularized lesion with early enhancement similar to that of pheochromocytoma [49].

On CT, adrenal carcinoma shows a heterogeneous appearance due to necrosis, calcifications and hemorrhage. After intravenous contrast injection, it demonstrates heterogeneous and mainly peripheral enhancement [49]. Invasion of adjacent structures such as kidney, inferior vena cava and splenic vessels are common as well as liver metastasis and retroperitoneal lymph nodal locations.

On MR, cortical carcinoma is hypointense on T1-weighted images, hyperintense on T2-weighted images, and there is strong and heterogeneous postcontrast enhancement with slow washout [65]. If there are hemorrhagic areas,they present hyperintense on T1-weighted images (Figure 8) [65]. Rarely, focal loss of signal intensity on out-of-phase images due to foci of intracytoplasmic fat may be observed [65].

Feminizing adrenal tumors are extremely rare malignant tumors with prevailing estrogen secretion and associated symptoms. The diagnosis is based on clinical features and hormonal assessment. CT may confirm the mass, but is not specific. Prognosis is generally poor. Virilizing adrenal tumors are also very rare, with few case reports presented in the literature.

CUSHING'S SYNDROME

Cushing's syndrome is a state of pathologic hypercortisolism as a result of excessive adrenocorticotropic hormone (ACTH) production, or autonomous adrenal production of cortisol. It is a potentially life-threatening disorder, and is associated with hypertension, diabetes, coagulopathy, cardiovascular disease, infections and fractures. Mortality may still be high even after hypercortisolism has been treated. Establishing the correct diagnosis as early as possible is important to prevent morbidity and residual disease [66]. Clinical features suggesting the syndrome include fatigue or hypomania, growth retardation in children, a variety of psychiatric and cognitive symptoms, metabolic syndromes including glucose intolerance, diabetes, infertility, hypogonadism, muscle weakness, abnormal adipose in dorsocervical and supraclavicular areas, skin manifestations, hypertension, decreased bone density and fractures. Symptoms that occur at an unusual age (fractures, hypertension, failure to progress in puberty, memory and cognitive changes) are more likely to reflect underlying hypercortisolism. Progressive accumulation of features over time is also more suggestive of the disease than a few features at one point in time. However, because some or many of these symptoms are already common among the general population to reach the correct diagnosis, the clinicians must evaluate the duration of signs and symptoms, and how fast these symptoms proceed as well as the appropriate biochemical testing. Once the diagnosis has been made, the cause has to be identified as the ideal treatment is surgical resection of the abnormal tumor/tissue. In cases where surgery is not possible, or there is recurrent or metastatic disease, medical therapy is preferred to normalize cortisol levels [66].

Cushing's syndrome should be considered in a patient presenting with signs and symptoms suggestive of the syndrome, which cannot be explained in another way [66]. Because many of the features may cluster under a single diagnosis, it is very important for subspecialists to look for features outside of their subject matter expertise, to avoid missing the diagnosis.

As an example, if a young woman presents with recent onset of hirsutism, acne and oligomenorrhea, and has also additional symptoms, such as depression, easy bruising and memory problems, Cushing's syndrome should be included in the differential diagnosis along with polycystic ovarian disease because the non-gynecologic symptoms suggest the former diagnosis. If wide purple striae or proximal muscle weakness are also present in such a patient, the diagnosis of Cushing's syndrome is more likely.

In another example, the presence of weight gain, new onset of hypertension and prediabetes in a 50 year old man with a family history of hypertension and diabetes, who lives a sedentary life would suggest essential hypertension and familial diabetes as likely diagnoses. However, if there is also history of recent pulmonary embolism, or if the patient has also multiple vertebral fractures, then the differential diagnosis should also include Cushing's syndrome. When signs and symptoms such as osteoporosis, fractures or hypertension are encountered in young adults, or when a patient presents with severe signs and symptoms of the syndrome that occur within a short time interval (such as a few months), or when more and more signs and symptoms appear progressively over a period of time, Cushing's syndrome should be considered. In another example, the diagnosis of Cushing's syndrome should be considered in a patient with weight gain within the last 2 or 3 months, who suffers from muscle weakness and impaired cognition because of hypokalemia. Conversely, weight gain over a longer time period, mood changes, hypertension and diabetes should also prompt evaluation for Cushing's syndrome. Exogenous exposure to glucocorticoid(s) may also cause Cushing's syndrome. Glucocorticoids are present in prescribed medicines for use via the oral, topical, rectal, or inhaled routes. Also, injections for joint or back pain, or a variety of non-prescription topical medications and "tonics" may also contain potent glucocorticoids. "Fair skin" preparations used to lighten skin may contain potent glucocorticoids that are absorbed systemically and cause exogenous Cushing's syndrome. Some products sold in the United Kingdom, Africa and India have been documented to contain unlabeled glucocorticoid [66]. In Asia, there exists concern about the association of the use of skin bleaching cream with possible development of Cushing's syndrome because of lack of information about the steroid content of these creams [66].It is recommended to measure synthetic steroids (dexamethasone, clobetasol, betamethasone, fluocinolone, and hydrocortisone) in blood or urine of Cushingoid individuals using these products. Even Cushingoid patients using traditional herbal medicals should be evaluated accordingly as these medicals may also contain glucocorticoids [66].

Screening Tests for Cushing's Syndrome

Endocrine Society guidelines recommend the use of at least two of three different screening tests: 24-hour urine free cortisol (UFC) excretion, late night/bedtime salivary cortisol levels and the 1 mg overnight dexamethasone suppression test (DST; or alternatively the 2 mg 2-day DST) [66]. Each of these screening tests reflects different physiologic abnormalities in Cushing's syndrome: high integrated daily cortisol production (UFC), loss of bedtime salivary or serum cortisol nadir, and impaired response to glucocorticoid negative feedback. Therefore, these tests are complimentary and a minimum of two tests should be used. The results should not contradict each other. The result of each cortisol screening test (saliva, serum, urine) is considered normal if it falls within the normal reference range; cortisol values 8 hours after administration of

1 mg dexamethasone at 2,300 to 2,400 hours should normally be less than 1.8 μg/dL (50 nmol/L). Cortisol may be measured by an immunoassay (e.g., radioimmunoassay [RIA]) or a structurally-based assay (e.g., high performance liquid chromatography or mass spectrometry [MS/ MS]). Structural-based assays are specific for cortisoland do not show cross-reactivity inherent to antibody-based assays. Therefore the upper limit of normal for the structural assays is lower than that of the antibody-based assays. However because of their inherent cross-reactivity immunoassays enable detection of mild cases of CS [67] as well as exposure to non-cortisol exogenous glucocorticoids. Each test has its drawbacks, so that the choice of tests should be tailored for each patient, to minimize false positive and false negative results [68]. Some patients with increased cortisol and features consistent with Cushing's syndrome such as weight gain, depression or hypertensionmay be seen in the general population. This overlap has been termed as "pseudo-Cushing's syndrome," and may lead to misdiagnosis of Cushing's syndrome. In these patients, the underlying condition associated with non-pathologic hypercortisolism can be treated. Generally, these patients do not progress to overt Cushing's syndrome over time with normalization of cortisol levels.

Recent Changes in the Management of Cushings's Syndrome

General Considerations

Cushing's syndrome (CS) is associated with increased morbidity and mortality, mainly caused by the coagulopathy (myocardial infarction, stroke, pulmonary embolism) or infection [66] and the consequences of hypertension and diabetes, all likely induced by an excess in cortisol [66]. Thus, the goal of treatment is to normalize cortisol levels or its action at the receptors, and to treat any comorbid condition. Treatment of comorbidities may take some time after cortisol levels are reduced, so each comorbidity should be treated specifically (e.g., with antihypertensives or insulin), while the treatment of CS continues [69].

Causes of Cushing's Syndrome

The causes of Cushing's syndrome can be divided into disorders of ACTH excess (either from a pituitary or non-pituitary [ectopic] tumor) and disorders of ACTH-independent primary adrenal overproduction of cortisol (adenoma, carcinoma, or bilateral macronodular/micronodular hyperplasias), in which plasma ACTH levels are low or undetectable. Once the Cushing's syndrome is diagnosed, levels of ACTH are determined as a first step to identify the cause. Patients with low/undetectable ACTH levels should undergo CT and/or MR examination to look for unilateral adrenal masses with adjacent and contralateral atrophy or bilateral disease. Patients with normal or elevated ACTH levels should undergo additional testing, including pituitary MRI, inferior petrosal sinus sampling, corticotropin releasing hormone, and/or 8 mg dexamethasone suppression [70]. Optimal treatment of Cushing's syndrome necessitates detection and subsequent removal of abnormal ACTH- or cortisol-producing tissue/tumor which leads to decrease of hypercortisolism and preservation of the normal hypothalamic-pituitary-adrenal axis.

Alternatives to Surgical Removal of Tumor

Patients with adrenal adenomas or with other primary adrenal causes of CS are ideally treated by surgical removal of the lesion(s) leading almost always to permanent cure. However, patients with adrenal cancer and those with ACTH-dependent disorders may have locally invasive disease or distant metastases. However patients with ectopic or pituitary ACTH-secreting tumors may remain occult after imaging or at transsphenoidal exploration, respectively. So in cases where the tumor cannot be fully resected or identified other alternatives must be considered to normalize cortisol including blockage of cortisol action at its receptor with a glucocorticoid antagonist, inhibition of cortisol synthesis with a steroidogenesis inhibitor or mitotane, or removal of both adrenal glands. Medical treatments aiming the hypophysis include somatostatin or dopamine analogs to reduce ACTH production.

Steroidogenesis Inhibitors and Glucocorticoid Antagonists

Metyrapone (11β-hydroxylase), ketoconazole (side chain cleavage, 17-hydroxylase and 17,20-lyase, 11β-hydroxylase and aldosterone synthase), and mitotane (11β-hydroxylase and cholesterol side chain cleavage; with additional cytotoxic effects at high doses) inhibit adrenal steroidogenesis at various enzymatic steps. Their use as monotherapy has been shown to be effective in about 50% of patients [66], though their combined use is also common, especially in hypercortisolism.

Mifepristone is a U.S. Food and Drug Administration-approved glucocorticoid receptor antagonist used for the treatment of hyperglycemia in patients with Cushing's syndrome [71].

The results of some studies have suggested that combination therapy rather than monotherapy should be used in the setting of severe hypercortisolism, which may be life-threatening as it may lead to infections and thrombotic phenomena [66].

To conclude, a careful history, judicious choice of screening tests and observation over time may enable to correctly diagnose Cushing's syndrome. When surgical resection of the causal tumor/tissue is not possible, medical treatment to reduce cortisol production may be life-saving.

SUBCLINICAL CUSHING'S SYNDROME (SCS)

SCS (also called subclinical autonomous glucocorticoid hypersecretion) is seen in patients with an incidentally detected adrenal adenoma. Two distinct criteria have to be met to make the diagnosis. First, there should be no signs and symptoms of Cushing syndrome in the patient as assessed by an experienced clinician, second, the adrenal mass should be detected incidentally at an examination performed for an unrelated reason. The likely cause of this cortisol hypersecretion is commonly a cortical adenoma, while adrenocortical carcinoma (ACC) is another less-likely possibility [72]. Because of the vague clinical manifestations of SCS biochemical tests should be obtained in establishing a diagnosis.

Assessment of SCS by biochemical testing may be challenging. Cortisol secretion and activation of the HPA axis runs in a continuum from unmistakably hypoactive (i.e., adrenal incidentaloma) to normal to hyperactive. Therefore assigning arbitrary cutoff values for the numerous biochemical tests assessing cortisol secretion and the HPA axis may lead to failure to identify the disease when such cutoffs are set too stringently, especially in patients with adrenal incidentaloma. Moreover, the circadian rhythm of cortisol secretion, which persists even in disease states, lowers the reproducibility of certain biochemical test results.

Dexamethasone-Suppression Testing

Dexamethasone-suppression testing (DST) is the key test used to diagnose SCS as it can evaluate mild elevations in cortisol secretion. Dexamethasone is used because as an endogenous steroid it does not cross-react with either immunologic or chemical assays for cortisol. In individuals with overt or subclinical corticotropin (adrenocorticotropic hormone [ACTH])-dependent hypercortisolism dexamethasone administration suppresses the HPA axis and results in reduction of cortisol secretion. 1 mg overnight DST is performed commonly for the diagnosis of SCS [72]. The NIH and the American Association of Clinical Endocrinologists/American Association of Endocrine Surgeons recommend the standard cut-off of 5 mg/dL as the upper limit of normal for serum cortisol following DST in patients with adrenal incidentaloma [73]. This cutoff yields a specificity over 90%whereas the sensitivity is poor at this cutoff as most normal individuals have cortisol levels suppressed to below 1 mg/dL after overnight DST [72]. Therefore, a cutoff of 3 mg/dL has also been widely recommended, which may minimize false-positive results while maintaining a modestly increased sensitivity [72].

The 2-day, 2-mg DST (sometimes referred to as low-dose DST) is preferred in patients with alcoholism, diabetes, or psychiatric disorders as it appears to be more accurate in these patients, though the reason is not known [74].

Corticotropin (Adrenocorticotropic Hormone)

In ACTH-independent hypercortisolism as in cases of most cortisol-secreting adrenal tumors serum ACTH levels are suppressed below 10 pg/mL. However, the specificity of low ACTH levels alone in diagnosing SCS is around 38% to 60% and furthermore ACTH levels can be normal even in ACTH-independent hypercortisolism, so ACTH alone is an unreliable tool in diagnosing SCS necessitating additional testing [72]. However, in patients with known SCS who have bilateral or diffuse adrenal enlargement ACTH testing can be used to rule out occult pituitary or ectopic ACTH-dependent hypercortisolism as the cause rather than AI. In such a case ACTH is not suppressed beyond 10 pg/mL. In uncertain cases (i.e., ACTH >10 pg/mL but <20 pg/mL), CRH stimulation testing can be performed. ACTH-dependent SCS can be excluded if the ACTH level is lower than 30 pg/mL after CRH stimulation [72].

Dehydroepiandrosterone Sulfate

Dehydroepiandrosterone (DHEA) is the most abundant circulating steroid hormone in humans. Reduction in DHEA sulfate (DHEA-S) levels is a frequent finding in AI. But because DHEA-S also decreases with age low DHEA-S serum concentration cannot be used as a useful diagnostic test for SCS [72].

Urinary Free Cortisol

Ordinarily, cortisol secretion has a circadian rhythms, with serum levels reaching their lowest point at midnight and then peaking approximately 1 hour after waking. Measurement of urinary free cortisol (UFC) provides a direct and reliable assessment of cortisol secretion [72].However, UFC can be affected by a number of patient factors and there is lack of reliable reference in laboratories for UFC measurement UFC alone has limited applicability in SCS screening, and should be combined with another modality for the diagnosis of SCS.

Midnight Cortisol

Higher than normal cortisol levels at the time of the usual midnight nadir suggests an abnormality in the regular circadian rhythm, and indicates hypercortisolism. However, besides its cumbersome applicability for the patients, Midnight Cortisol levels have also low sensitivity to diagnose SCS and are therefore mainly used as confirmatory testing.

Approach to SCS Diagnosis in Adrenal Incidentaloma

In a patient with newly discovered AI, there is no single biochemical test that delivers adequate accuracy to reliably diagnose SCS. Studies conducted on patients with suspicious SCS who present with osteopenia, hypertension or diabetes mellitus biochemical testing for SCS was conducted and CRH, midnight cortisol testing, UFC, ACTH, and overnight DST (with a 5 mg/dL cutoff for a positive test) have been evaluated where only DST reached 90% in specificity [76]. Overnight 1-mg DST offers excellent sensitivity when using a low cutoff for positivity, but with a significant decline in specificity. Use of a combination of overnight 1-mg DST (with a 3 mg/dL cutoff), elevated UFC above the normal limit, and serum ACTH of less than 10 pg/mL has been suggested which yielded sensitivity and specificity exceeding 60% and showed an accuracy of 75.8% for predicted SCS-related complications when abnormalities in at least 2 of the 3 tests was considered diagnostic of SCS [77].

A thorough history and physical examination must be performed as well, and correlated with any findings. In patients with equivocal testing results serial measurements at regular intervals and addition of adjunctive tests, such as DHEA-S is recommended. It is to be noted that all treatments should be tailored on an individual-based strategy as there are still no widely accepted standard diagnostic criteria for SCS.

Adrenal Scintigraphy

Patients with SCS have minimal alterations in their biochemical profiles. Utilization of iodocholesterol scintigraphy has been studied and yielded inconsistent results to diagnose SCS. Therefore, adrenal scintigraphy has not gained general acceptance, and therefore is only offered in a few select institutions worldwide.

Indications for Surgery in SCS

There are mainly 2 clinical options for patients with SCS: Patient monitoring and surgical resection. Some studies conducting patient surveillance reported mild disease progression over 25.5 months monitoring while others showed progression to overt Cushing's syndrome in 12.5% of patients over 1 year follow-up [78].

Adrenalectomy has been proved to ameliorate the biochemical abnormalities associated with SCS, but its long-term effects are not clear yet [72]. Adrenalectomy has been demonstrated to decrease the cardiovascular risk factors and to reverse the comorbidities associated with SCS [79]. In general, in biochemically proven or suspected SCS or with a lesion greater than 4 cm surgical resection by an experienced surgeon is recommended, given the low morbidity and mortality associated with either laparoscopic, or more recently, posterior retroperitoneoscopic adrenalectomy. Patients should receive perioperative glucocorticoid supplementation because of the risk of acute Addisonian crisis [72]. Given the subclinical nature of SCS, it remains extremely difficult to accurately determine clinical improvement; nevertheless, patients should be monitored and continued on a short steroid course until they have a proven intact HPA axis according to previously established protocols [72].

CONGENITAL ADRENAL HYPERPLASIA

Congenital adrenal hyperplasia (CAH) is associated with deficiency of steroid 21-hydroxylase. It is the most common inborn error in adrenal function and the most common cause of adrenal insufficiency in the pediatric age group. In most patients with CAH, 21-hydroxylase deficiency results in decrease in both cortisol and aldosterone production while increased production of adrenal androgen is seen as a side effect. As a result of the lack of the vital hormones cortisol and aldosterone, adrenal insufficiency may ensue which may be fatal if untreated. Excess androgen production causes ambiguous genitaliain females along with various endocrinologic, gynecologic, and reproductive complications. Males with CAH may present with iso-sexual precocity, reproductive and endocrine disorders, most notably with testicular adrenal rest tumors and oligospermia [80].

Prenatal and Neonatal Diagnosis

CAH is a monogenic autosomal recessive disease caused by mutations or deletions in*CYP21A2*, the gene encoding steroid 21-hydroxylase [81].The diagnosis of classic 21-hydroxylase deficiency (21OHD) is made when very high serum levels of 17-hydroxyprogesterone (17OHP), the normal substrate for 21-hydroxylase (17OHP) are detected in blood. Neonatal screening for 21OHD is an approved part of the neonatal screening program in many countries, including the USA. The screening test for 17OHP is measured using a filter paper blood sample obtained by a heel puncture preferably between two and four days after birth. The assay used in most programs is a fluoroimmunoassay (DELFIA). Adrenal ultrasonography is another potential adjunctive test for CAH in neonates with atypical genitalia and/or life-threatening salt loss, when the diagnosis is equivocal based upon other testing.

Newborn screening decreases infant morbidity and mortality associated with adrenal insufficiency because of earlier diagnosis and treatment [80]. Genotyping is most often performed when the hormonal diagnosis is in question or when genetic counseling is indicated [80]. Extracting fetal DNA from the maternal circulation at as early as 5 to 6 weeks showed promising results for earlier anticipatory guidance [82].

The primary aim in treating classic CAH is to decrease excess adrenal androgen, CRH and ACTH secretion and to substitute the deficient glucocorticoid cortisol and mineralocorticoid aldosterone.

Proper treatment of hyperandrogenemia with cortisol will allow normalization of growth, sex maturation and later reproductive function while replacement of aldosterone will help maintain normal serum electrolytes, extracellular fluid volume and plasma renin activity. Once the diagnosis has been established in the infant daily oral medications, including glucocorticoids, mineralocorticoids, and salt supplements are supplied after adequate titration according to blood levels of adrenal steroids, plasma renin activity, and electrolytes which are measured periodically, along with annual bone age x-rays. Supplemental salt is not required in older children and adults whose diets already contain more than enough sodium. Growth rate and weight gain should also be monitored regularly since overtreatment or under treatment may be associated with inappropriate growth. The preferred treatment in children and adults is hydrocortisone, the least potent glucocorticoid with a short half-life given in two or three daily doses [80].

During major stress conditions such as surgery, or serious illness, patients with CAH require larger or more frequent doses (or both) of glucocorticoids and additional fluids. Failure to provide glucocorticoids during these stress instances may lead to high mortality rates [83].

Women with CAH most often present with female core gender identity and behavior despite exposure to prenatal androgens [80].Fertility and fecundity are reduced in both men and women with CAH compared with controls. For women with CAH, adequate control of adrenal hormones, particularly follicular phase progesterone, is key in both conception and fetal retention [80]. Pregnant women with classic CAH should receive adjustments to steroid doses and careful fetal monitoring. Due to an efficient placental aromatase enzyme system female fetuses cannot be easily virilized by transplacental passage of maternal androgens.

Mineralocorticoid Excess Syndromes

The syndrome of apparent mineralocorticoid excess (AME), a genetic disorder, and chronic ingestion of licorice or licorice-like compounds can result in findings seen in primary aldosteronism: hypertension, hypokalemia, metabolic alkalosis, and low plasma renin activity. However, unlike elevated plasma aldosterone levels of primary aldosteronism levels of aldosterone are low in these disorders.

Renal mineralocorticoid receptors bind aldosterone and cortisol with similar affinity. Although the plasma concentration of cortisol is approximately 100-fold higher than aldosterone, activation of mineralocorticoid receptors by cortisol is normally limited due to its conversion to inactive cortisone at the sites of aldosterone binding sites (such as renal cortical collecting tubules)by the enzyme 11-beta-hydroxysteroid dehydrogenase type 2 (11-beta-HSD2) [84]. This inactive cortisone does not bind to the mineralocortiocoid receptors. In patients with AME, there is a mutation in the 11-beta-HSD2 gene on chromosome 16 with resulting impaired activity of 11-beta-HSD2 enzyme, which is controlled by the gene. Other mutations in other genes have also been described some with partial inhibitions on 11-beta-HSD2 enzyme activity [85]. As a result increased levels of active cortisol act on mineralocorticoid receptors causing signs of hyperaldosteronism at the presence of low aldosterone levels.

Licorice ingestion also has a similar effect because of a compound in licorice (glycyrrhetinic acid) that inhibits the enzyme [86].

By somewhat different mechanisms, hypersecretion of cortisol can also induce an excess mineralocorticoid state in patients with ectopic ACTH syndrome [87].

The Syndrome of Apparent Mineralocorticoid Excess (AME)

Clinical Manifestations

The syndrome of AME is an autosomal recessive genetic disorder and is a rare form of severe juvenile hypertension [88]. Clinical manifestations are low birth weight, failure to thrive, muscle weakness, onset of severe hypertension in early childhood with extensive target organ damage, hypercalciuria, nephrocalcinosis and renal failure. All of the findings of primary aldosteronism (hypertension, hypokalemia, metabolic alkalosis, and low plasma renin activity) are present, except for the low plasma aldosterone concentration. Chronic hypokalemia may lead to nephrogenic diabetes insipidus and subsequent polyuria [88].

Diagnosis

The biochemical abnormalities suggesting the diagnosis include:

- Hypokalemia
- Metabolic alkalosis
- Low plasma renin activity
- Low plasma aldosterone levels

The UFC to urinary free cortisone ratio as measured on a 24-hour urine collection is a sensitive diagnostic test [89]. Normally, urinary free cortisone levels outnumber UFC levels by a ratio of approximately 0.3 to 0.5.In patients with AME, the urinary free cortisone levels are very low or undetectable, so the ratio of cortisol to cortisone is 5 in children, 18 in adults [89].

Differential Diagnosis

The presenting symptoms and signs of AME are similar to those of primary aldosteronism, but the plasma aldosterone concentration is low.

Licorice ingestion and ectopic ACTH syndrome can have similar biochemical findings as of AME. However, assessment of UFC and cortisone levels allows differentiation of these disorders [90]:

- With licorice ingestion, urinary cortisone is only modestly decreased, and thus there is mild elevation of the ratio.
- Ectopic ACTH production may result in a similarly elevated urinary free cortisol to cortisone ratio, however since there is no associated enzymatic defect urinary cortisone is also elevated along with urinary cortisol which contrasts to the very low levels of urinary free cortisone excretion in the syndrome of AME.

AME must also be distinguished from other rare causes of mineralocorticoid excess in which aldosterone levels are reduced, including Liddle's syndrome (due to a gain-of-function mutation in the collecting tubule sodium channel), deoxycorticosterone-secreting tumors, deficiency in the 5-reductase enzyme (leading to defective conversion and thus persistently high levels of cortisol), and two forms of congenital adrenal hyperplasia [80]. Urinary cortisol metabolites are normal in the first two disorders.

Treatment

The main goal of treatment of the syndrome of AME should aim to reduce endogenous cortisol production or block the mineralocorticoid receptor. Potassium repletion, if required for hypokalemiaand antagonism of mineralocorticoid effect with amiloride or eplerenone should be tried. If mineralocorticoid antagonism is not effective or not tolerated. Dexamethasone in doses of 1.5 to 2 mg/day may be given to suppress ACTH and reduce endogenous cortisol production without activating the mineralocorticoid receptor. However, dexamethasone does not correct the hypokalemia and hypertension in all patients and its long-term use may have adverse effects [84]. Normalization of the plasma potassium concentration seems to be a reasonable end point of treatment. A thiazide is indicated if hypercalciuria or nephrocalcinosis is present [84].

Licorice Ingestion

Chronic ingestion of licorice or licorice-like compounds (such as carbenoxolone) causes a syndrome with findings similar to those with the syndrome of AME: hypertension, hypokalemia, metabolic alkalosis, low plasma renin activity and low plasma aldosterone levels [91].

Licorice contains a steroid, glycyrrhetinic acid, that inhibits (both competitively and by reducing gene expression) 11-beta-HSD2, the same enzyme that is deficient in AME. The diagnosis is typically based upon the biochemical abnormalities and an elicited history of licorice ingestion. Cessation of licorice ingestion (or other source of glycyrrhetinic acid) is usually the only treatment necessary. Hypokalemia may be initially treated with potassium supplements or a potassium-sparing diuretic, however such treatment should not be extended beyond one week after the effects of licorice have subsided.

Ectopic ACTH Syndrome

Increased levels of cortisole can cause excess mineralocorticoid effect in Cushing's syndrome due to ectopic ACTH release (most commonly arising from small cell carcinoma of the lung), by one of the following ways:

- Excessive cortisol hypersecretion may exceed the metabolic capacity of 11-beta-HSD2 [87].
- Extremely high circulating levels of ACTH may inhibit 11-beta-HSD2.

- Hypersecretion of non-aldosterone mineralocorticoids, such as deoxycorticosterone and corticosterone.

The diagnosis of the ectopic ACTH syndrome is suggested by hypokalemia, the demonstration of markedly increased 24-hour urinary free cortisol excretion, and elevated serum ACTH.

PRIMARY ALDOSTERONISM (CONN'S SYNDROME)

Primary aldosteronism (PA) presents with hypertension and hypokalemia with frequently normal levels of potassium. It is caused by non-suppressible hypersecretion of aldosterone.

The most common subtypes of primary aldosteronism are:

- Aldosterone-producing adenomas (APAs)
- Bilateral idiopathic hyperaldosteronism (IHA; bilateral adrenal hyperplasia)

Less common causes are:

- Familial hyperaldosteronism types I to IV
- Unilateral adrenal hyperplasia
- Pure aldosterone-producing adrenocortical carcinomas
- Ectopic aldosterone-producing tumors

A multicenter study revealed that in 5-10% of all hypertensive patients PA is the causative etiology as detected by plasma aldosterone to renin ratio [92].

The presence of the triad of hypertension, unexplained hypokalemia, and metabolic alkalosis in any patient should raise the suspicion of primary mineralocorticoid excess [93], although most patients with PA are normokalemic and very few normotensive (primarily in young adult females).

Before making the diagnosis of PA etiologies causing secondary hyperaldosteronism such as heavy vomiting, diuretic therapy, and Bartter syndrome should be ruled out as PRA and plasma renin concentration (PRC) are increased in these cases rather than suppressed as in PA. Normokalemia is invariably present in patients with the rare genetic disorder glucocorticoid-remediable aldosteronism (familial hyperaldosteronism).

There is higher rate of cardiovascular morbidity and mortality associated with compared with age- and sex-matched patients with primary hypertension [94]. Therefore correct diagnosis of PA is important as treatment of PA results in reversal or improvement of the hypertension and decrease of the cardiovascular risk.

The Diagnosis of Primary Aldosteronism

Plasma renin activity (PRA) or plasma renin concentration (PRC) and plasma aldosterone concentration (PAC) are measured from the morning blood sample that has been obtained from ambulatory patient groups with a high prevalence of PA.

In PA, PRA or PRC is suppressed (PRA <1 ng/mL/hour; PRC less than the lower limit of reference range) and the PAC is inappropriately high for the PRA (typically >15 ng/dL [416 pmol/L], but as low as 10 ng/dL [277 pmol/L]). However, definitive diagnosis of PA should be confirmed by demonstrating elevated levels of aldosterone. Aldosterone suppression testing is also needed which includes oral administration of sodium chloride and measurement of urine aldosterone excretion or intravenous sodium chloride loading and measurement of PAC. In a patient with spontaneous hypokalemia, undetectable PRA or PRC or PAC ≥20 ng/dL (555 pmol/L) PA is the only possible diagnosis with no further testing necessary.

Once the diagnosis of primary aldosteronism has been established, a unilateral aldosterone-producing adenoma, or rarely, carcinoma, must be distinguished from bilateral hyperplasia. This is important since the treatment options are different for the two disorders. The Endocrine Society 2016 clinical practice guidelines [95] recommend testing of patients with hypertension and spontaneous or low-dose, diuretic-induced hypokalemia. Patients with the following signs and symptoms should also be tested even if they are normokalemic:

- Severe hypertension (>150 mmHg systolic or >100 mmHg diastolic) or drug-resistant hypertension (defined as suboptimally controlled hypertension on a combination of antihypertensives including an adrenergic inhibitor, vasodilator, and diuretic)
- Hypertension with adrenal incidentaloma
- Hypertension with sleep apnea
- Hypertension and a family history of early-onset hypertension or cerebrovascular accident at a young age (<40 years)
- All hypertensive first-degree relatives of patients with primary aldosteronism

The PRA and PRC are typically very low in patients with primary aldosteronism, usually less than 1 ng/mL per hour (0.2778 ng/L per sec) for PRA and usually undetectable or below the lower limit of normal for PRC [96]. On the other hand, increased PRA or PRC in a hypokalemic hypertensive patient is most often due to diuretic therapy, renovascular or malignant hypertension, or, rarely, a renin-secreting tumor.

The PAC is usually >15 ng/dL (416 pmol/L), but may be as low as 10 ng/dL (277 pmol/L).The mean value for the PAC/PRA ratio in normal subjects and patients with primary hypertension is 4 to 10, compared with more than 30 to 50 in most patients with primary aldosteronism [96]. PRA and PRC are low in a significant number of patients with primary hypertension, but a high PAC (typically >15 ng/dL [416 pmol/L]) and an abnormally high ratio are rare.

In general, a PAC/PRA ratio greater than 20 is considered suspicious for primary aldosteronism although there is a high variation in cutoff values making the PAC/PRA ratio unfavorable for case-detection. Thus, the paired random PAC and PRA (or PRC) are preferred for diagnosis.

Most antihypertensive medications can be continued however certain drugs may cause difficulty in interpreting data from patients tested for presence of PA. Mineralocorticoid receptor antagonists such as spironolactone and eplerenone block aldosterone from activating the receptor, resulting sequentially in sodium loss, a decrease in plasma volume, and an elevation in PRA, which will reduce the utility of the PAC/PRA ratio. These drugs should be discontinued until after the evaluation is completed. However if PRA is suppressed and the patients are hypokalemic these agents can be administered during testing. Amiloride and triamterene do not interfere with testing. Angiotensin-converting enzyme (ACE) inhibitors, angiotensin receptor blockers (ARBs), and direct renin inhibitors could potentially elevate PRC and have variable effects on PRA in patients with primary aldosteronism. In a patient taking one of these agents a PRA < 1ng/mL/hour or low PRC is strongly suggestive of PA whereas a PRA > 1ng/mL/hour does not rule out PA.

Other Causes of Hypertension and Hypokalemia

Secondary Hyperaldosteronism

Secondary hyperaldosteronism should be considered when both the PRA (and PRC) and PAC are increased and the PAC/PRA ratio is <10. In this setting, hypersecretion of renin leads sequentially to increased angiotensin II and then increased aldosterone secretion.

Causes of Secondary Hyperaldosteronism

Diuretic therapy in a hypokalemic hypertensive patient may lead to increased PRA or PRC. Less common causes include renovascular or malignant hypertension, Cushing's syndrome, certain forms of congenital adrenal hyperplasia, Liddle's syndrome, and rare renin-secreting tumors.

Cushing's syndrome (CS) may lead to hypokalemia due in part to the overproduction of (ACTH)-dependent compounds such as deoxycorticosterone, corticosterone, and cortisol. However, the associated hypertension in this disorder can usually be related to CS by the classic signs and symptoms of CS.

The degree of ACTH and cortisol hypersecretion (and therefore the frequency of hypokalemia) is much higher in the ectopic ACTH syndrome than with a pituitary adenoma.

Patients with renin-secreting tumors are typically young and have severe hypertension and hypokalemia. CT is usually diagnostic and surgical resection is considered to be curative.

Liddle's syndrome is a rare autosomal dominant disorder in which there is increase in sodium and often potassium reabsorption in the collecting tubules.

Nonaldosterone Mineralocorticoid Excess

The combination of suppressed PRA or PRC and a low plasma or urinary aldosterone value in a patient with hypertension and hypokalemia may indicate the presence of some nonaldosterone mineralocorticoid. This can occur in the following settings:

- Some types of congenital adrenal hyperplasia (deficiencies of 11-beta-hydroxylase or 17-alpha-hydroxylase) cause hypertension and hypokalemia because of hypersecretion of deoxycorticosterone. Familial cortisol resistance has a similar presentation.
- Chronic licorice root ingestion, AME, and severe cases of CS, in which cortisol acts as the primary mineralocorticoid. In CS, there may also be hypersecretion of other glucocorticoids such as deoxycorticosterone and corticosterone.
- A deoxycorticosterone-producing adrenal tumor, which can usually be detected by CT or MRI.

- Similar findings in the absence of mineralocorticoid excess are seen in Liddle's syndrome, with increased sodium reabsorption, potassium wasting, hypertension, and hypokalemia. Blocking the sodium channel with amiloride and triamterene can treat both the hypertension and hypokalemia.

24-Hour Urine Collection

There is no need for a 24-hour urine potassium measurement unless PRA is not suppressed, PAC is not elevated, or there is a clinical suspicion of surreptitious vomiting or laxative abuse.

Increased urinary potassium excretion with reduced serum potassium concentration is caused by a mineralocorticoid excess. When a 24-hour collection is obtained inappropriate potassium wasting is defined as more than 30 mEq/day in a patient with hypokalemia.

Elevated aldosterone excretion can also be seen (>12 mcg/day [33 nmol/day]) on a high-sodium diet (urine sodium excretion >200 mEq/day) being consistent with primary aldosteronism if the PRA is low. The rate of potassium excretion is best appreciated when the patient is on a high-sodium diet because the combination of increased distal flow and hypersecretion of aldosterone will maximize potassium losses. Sodium-induced hypokalemia is strongly suggestive of nonsuppressible hyperaldosteronism as potassium wasting does not occur in normal subjects where an increase in distal flow is balanced by reduced secretion of aldosterone.

However, aldosterone suppression testing is usually needed, and it can be performed with orally administered sodium chloride and measurement of urine aldosterone excretion or with intravenous sodium chloride loading and measurement of PAC [97].

Oral Sodium Loading

Oral sodium loading (5000 mg) over three days is recommended after hypertension and hypokalemia are controlled (hypokalemia suppresses aldosterone secretion). Since sodium loading increases kaliuresis and hypokalemia, serum potassium should be monitored and replaced as needed. On the third day of the diet, aldosterone, sodium, and creatinine are measured in serum and urine. Urine aldosterone excretion >12 mcg/24 hours (33 nmol/day) is consistent with hyperaldosteronism.

Saline Infusion Test

Suppression of endogenous aldosterone production can also be achieved by intravenous administration of 2 L of isotonic saline over four hours (from 8 AM to 12 PM). The patient should be seated to decrease false-negative results. The PAC will fall below 5 ng/dL (139 pmol/L) in normal subjects, whereas values above 10 ng/dL (277 pmol/L) are consistent with primary aldosteronism.

Once the diagnosis of primary aldosteronism has been established, differentiation of a unilateral aldosterone-producing adenoma (APA), or rarely, carcinoma, from bilateral hyperplasia (idiopathic hyperaldosteronism [IHA]) should be made as treatment is different. The Mayo Clinic uses an algorithm with adrenal CT and adrenal vein sampling (AVS) [97].

- In general, APA patients have higher aldosterone secretion rates, resulting in more severe hypertension, more profound hypokalemia (<3.2 mEq/L), and higher plasma (>25 ng/dL) and urinary (>30 mcg/24 hour) levels of aldosterone; these patients are also younger (<50 years) than those with IHA [97]. Somatic mutations in *KCNJ5*, *ATP1A1*, *ATP2B3*, *CTNNB1*, and *CACNA1D*are found in more than 50 percent of resected APAs [98].
- Bilateral adrenal hyperplasia presents with milder hyperaldosteronism and hypokalemia and accounts for approximately 60 percent of cases. Treatment includes use of a mineralocorticoid receptor antagonist.

Adrenal CT

CT should be preferred to MR as the initial study to assess the adrenal gland and to differentiate between an adenoma and hyperplasia or to rule out an adrenal carcinoma [99]. Non-contrast followed by contrast enhanced CT is required to identify characterize the adrenal mass.

- A unilateral, large (>4 cm) adrenal mass in a patient with primary aldosteronism may be suggestive of an adrenal carcinoma
- Adrenal hyperplasia may present with bilateral adrenal gland thickening or micronodular changes; however, it should be noted that patients with hyperplasia may also have normal-appearing adrenal glands on CT.
- When a solitary, hypodense, unilateral macroadenoma (>1 cm) and normal contralateral adrenal gland are found in patients of<35 years of age with vigorous primary aldosteronism, unilateral adrenalectomy should be considered whereas adrenal venous sampling should be preferred in patients with >35 years of age because of the possibility of a nonfunctioning adenoma.

Limitations of CT

CT findings may be unreliable in distinguishing between an adenoma and bilateral hyperplasia [41]. CT can also miss subcentimeter adrenal lesions so absence of a mass on CT does not exclude an adenoma which can be very small (e.g., <3 mm in diameter). Furthermore, demonstration of bilateral lesions is not necessarily diagnostic of hyperplasia (because some patients with an aldosteronoma in one adrenal gland have a nonfunctioning adrenal nodule in the other) [100]. Therefore, it is important to perform AVS in most patients to distinguish between unilateral and bilateral adrenal aldosterone hypersecretion.

Adrenal Vein Sampling (AVS)

Sampling should be performed by an experienced interventional radiologist. AVS is the criterion standard test to distinguish between unilateral adenoma and bilateral hyperplasia [101]. Unilateral disease is associated with a marked (usually fourfold greater than contralateral adrenal) increase in PAC on the side of the tumor, whereas there is little difference between the two sides in patients with bilateral hyperplasia [101].

Indications

AVS is performed in patients to plan unilateral adrenalectomy and is indicated in patients with primary aldosteronism who have

- Normal CT findings to confirm presence of unilateral disease
- Bilateral adrenal lesions on CT
- Unilateral adrenal lesion and patient age > 35 years [102].

Patients <35 years with a unilateral macroadenoma (>1cm and <2cm) do not need AVS. APA is more likely in patients who have spontaneous hypokalemia and marked elevations in aldosterone in blood (e.g., >30 ng/dL) or 24-hour urine collection (e.g., >30 mcg).

Procedure

Continuous cosyntropin infusion (50 mcg per hour started 30 minutes before sequential sampling of the adrenal veins and continued throughout the procedure) is recommended for the following reasons:

- To minimize stress-induced fluctuations in aldosterone secretion during nonsimultaneous AVS, which could potentially confound the interpretation of lateralization data.
- To maximize the gradient in cortisol from adrenal vein to inferior vena cava (IVC) and thus confirm successful sampling of the adrenal vein.
- To maximize the secretion of aldosterone from an APA.

Aldosterone and cortisol concentrations are measured in the blood from all right and left adrenal vein, and IVC). All of the blood samples should be assayed at 1:1, 1:10, and 1:50 dilutions; absolute values and accurate laboratory assays for cortisol and aldosterone are essential for successful interpretation of the AVS data.

Confirming Successful Catheterization

With cosyntropin infusion, the adrenal vein to IVC cortisol ratio is typically more than 10:1 [103]; a ratio of at least 5:1 is required to be confident that the adrenal veins were successfully catheterized.

Cortisol-Corrected Ratios

Dividing the right and left adrenal vein PAC by their respective cortisol concentrations corrects for the dilutional effect of the inferior phrenic vein flow into the left adrenal vein; these are termed "cortisol-corrected ratios."

- At Mayo Clinic, the mean cortisol-corrected aldosterone ratio (APA-side PAC/cortisol to normal adrenal PAC/cortisol) in patients with confirmed APA is 18:1 [103]. A a cutoff for the cortisol-corrected aldosterone ratio from high-side to low-side of more than 4:1 has been suggested to indicate unilateral aldosterone excess [103].
- In patients with presumed IHA, the mean cortisol-corrected aldosterone ratio is 1.8:1 (high-side to low-side); a ratio less than 3:1 is suggestive of bilateral aldosterone hypersecretion [103].

Thus, most patients with a unilateral source of aldosterone will have cortisol-corrected aldosterone lateralization ratios greater than 4. A ratio less than 3 suggests bilateral aldosterone hypersecretion [103]. Moreover, the contralateral aldosterone to cortisol ratio is less than the IVC aldosterone to cortisol ratio in a significant number of patients with surgically confirmed APA [103], indicative of suppression of aldosterone secretion by the noninvolved adrenal gland.

Results

AVS may be most useful when there is no adrenal abnormality on CT or when both adrenal glands are abnormal but asymmetric. One limitation to AVS is failure to collect adequate samples as the right adrenal vein is small and sometimes difficult to reach.

Familial Hyperaldosteronism

There are four other rare forms of familial hyperaldosteronism (FH) associated with adrenal hyperplasia:

- FH type I or glucocorticoid-remediable aldosteronism (GRA) due to a CYP11B1/CYP11B2 chimeric gene
- FH type II, caused by germline mutations in the chloride channel CLCN2
- FH type III, caused by germline mutations in the potassium channel subunit KCNJ5
- FH type IV, caused by germline mutations in the*CACNA1H*gene, which encodes the alpha subunit of an L-type voltage-gated calcium channel (Cav3.2)

There may be simultaneous cortisol cosecretion in larger APA's (e.g., ≥1.5 cm in diameter). Therefore, it is advisable to obtain a baseline serum dehydroepiandrosterone sulfate (DHEAS) and perform a 1 mg overnight dexamethasone suppression test and when cortisol cosecretion is documented, it is important to take adequate perioperative measures accordingly.

Pregnancy

Primary aldosteronism is uncommon in pregnancy. When present most patients have PA due to APA's [104]. PA can cause intrauterine growth retardation, preterm delivery, intrauterine fetal demise, and placental abruption.

Detection of PA in pregnant women is the same as in nonpregnant patients: morning blood sample for the assessment of aldosterone and plasma renin activity or renin concentration. Suppressed renin and an aldosterone level >10 ng/dL is a positive finding for primary aldosteronism. If spontaneous hypokalemia is present in the woman with high aldosterone (≥20 ng/dL) and suppressed renin, confirmatory testing is not needed. In the normokalemic woman with a positive case-detection test, confirmatory testing is needed with measurement of sodium and aldosterone in a 24-hour urine collection on an ambient sodium diet.

Characterization of the adrenal lesion with abdominal MRI without gadolinium is the test of choice. Adrenal CT, iodocholesterol scintigraphy, and adrenal vein sampling are not recommended in pregnancy.

Adrenal Insufficiency (AI)

Addison's disease (AD), also known as primary adrenal insufficiency, is a deficiency in the production of all hormones from adrenal cortex, i.e., glucocorticosteroids and mineral corticosteroids.

Primary AI affects more frequently women, and clinical manifestations can present at any age, although most often between 30 and 50 years [105].

In AD, the female: male ratio is 1.8 and adults of all ages are affected. It is estimated that AD affects 1 in 10 000 people in the UK, and throughout Europe. In developed countries the primary cause is autoimmune diseases and worldwide tuberculosis is the main cause. Other etiologies of AD are infections other than tubeculosis, genetic disorders, adrenal hemorrhage, bilateral adrenal metastases or infiltration, bilateral adrenalectomy and drug-induced [106].

There is a chronic gradual destruction of the adrenocortical tissue through cell-mediated or direct cytotoxic mechanisms in AD. At this early stage, there is high plasma renin activity and low aldosterone. With gradual loss of more adrenocortical tissue initially there is reduction to suboptimal baseline cortisol level with a maintained response to stress which in turn is impaired in time. At this stage, a minor stressor can precipitate an adrenal crisis. With further and almost complete destruction of the adrenocortical tissue even the basal cortisol secretion is low causing the clinical onset of symptoms of disease while there is an increased ACTH level due to the negative feedback. High ACTH leads to skin hyperpigmentation because its cleavage product alpha-MSH which is responsible for the pigmentation is also increased. In around one-half of patients with AD the presentation is acute with adrenal crisis which may be fatal. In the remainder of AD patients the presentation is chronic with vague and insidious symptoms in which case the diagnosis can be delayed [107].Adrenal crisis should be suspected in any patient with peripheral vascular collapse (vasodilatory shock), whether or not the patient is known to have AD. Likewise, isolated ACTH-deficiency which is rare should be considered in any patient with unexplained hypoglycemia or hyponatremia [106].

Secondary (pituitary) AI occurs more frequently than primary adrenal insufficiency. Its estimated prevalence is 150–280 per million and is more common in women than men. Affected patients are mostly diagnosed in the sixth decade of life. Causes of secondary AI are space-occupying lesions in the pituitary, pituitary trauma and genetic mutations related to the pituitary [108].

The most common cause of *tertiary (hypothalamic) AI* is chronic exogenous administration of synthetic glucocorticoids, which causes prolonged suppression of hypothalamic corticotropin-releasing hormone (CRH) secretion through negative feedback leading to decreased secretion of ACTH. Tumors, infections and trauma of the hypothalamus are other causes [108]. In secondary or tertiary adrenal insufficiency, the resultant ACTH deficiency leads to decreased secretion of cortisol and adrenal androgens, while mineralocorticoid production remains normal.

Common signs and symptoms of chronic AD are owing to deficient concentrations of all adrenocortical hormones (mineralocorticoids, glucocorticoids, adrenal androgens) and include general malaise, fatigue, weakness, anorexia, weight loss, nausea, vomiting, abdominal pain or diarrhea, which may alternate with constipation, hypotension, electrolyte abnormalities (hyponatremia, hyperkalemia, metabolic acidosis), hyperpigmentation, autoimmune manifestations (vitiligo), decreased axillary and pubic hair, and loss of libido and amenorrhea in women [108].

The clinical features of secondary or tertiary AI are similar to those of AD with the exception of skin hyperpigmentation because the secretion of ACTH is not increased. Also, dehydration and hyperkalemia are absent as production of mineralocorticoids by the zona glomerulosa is mostly preserved. As a result hypotension is less prominent. However, hyponatremia and increased intravascular volume may be seen due to "inappropriate" increase in vasopressin secretion. Hypoglycemia is more common in secondary adrenal insufficiency possibly due to concomitant growth hormone insufficiency and in isolated ACTH deficiency. Clinical manifestations of a pituitary or hypothalamic tumor and associated symptoms and signs of deficiency of other anterior pituitary hormones may also be present [108].

The relative or functional adrenal insufficiency that is seen during critical illness as a result of subnormal corticosteroid production during without associated structural defects in the HPA axis is a different entity and should be distinguished from the primary AI (AD).There is currently no consensus on the diagnostic criteria for this entity.

Diagnosis

Diagnosis of AI is made by demonstrating inappropriately low levels of cortisol, followed by the determination of the cortisol deficiency whether it is primary or secondary. The clinical diagnosis of chronic adrenal insufficiency is often more difficult than that of acute adrenal insufficiency as the signs and symptoms in chronic AD may be confusing. For instance, hyperpigmentation is not necessarily present in all AD patients and is always absent in secondary (pituitary) and tertiary (hypothalamic) AI.

Endocrine evaluation is indicated to confirm the diagnosis even in obvious cases and to determine the type of AI and its cause. However, therapy should be initiated before the diagnosis is established in an acutely ill patient with possible adrenal crisis.

The progression of adrenal insufficiency is often gradual and may go undetected until an illness or other stress precipitates an adrenal crisis. Adrenal crisis is most commonly precipitated in the chronic course of AD when a major stress, serious infection, adrenal infarction or hemorrhage intervenes. The main precipitating factor of adrenal crisis is mineralocorticoid deficiency. Unmet mineralocorticoid demands during glucocorticoid therapy may also lead to adrenal crisis. Hypotensive shock is the main manifestation of adrenal crisis, but non-specific and vague abdominal symptoms may also be seen.

Laboratory Diagnosis

Basal Morning Serum Cortisol Concentrations

The diagnosis of AI is based first on the demonstration of inappropriately low cortisol secretion. Then, it should be determined if the cortisol deficiency is caused by a ACTH-deficiency or independent from it, and in ACTH-independent cases mineralocorticoid secretion should also be evaluated. And finally, a treatable cause of the primary disorder should be sought if any present [109].

Serum cortisol concentrations are normally highest in the early morning hours (06:00h – 08:00h), ranging between 10 – 20 mcg/dL (275 – 555 nmol/L) than at other times of the day. Early morning serum cortisol levels of less than 3 μg/dL (80 nmol/L) are strongly suggestive of adrenal insufficiency [110], while values below 10 μg/dL (275 nmol/L) make the diagnosis likely. Simultaneous measurements of cortisol and ACTH concentrations confirm in most cases the diagnosis of primary adrenal insufficiency. A morning cortisol above 18 mcg/dL is reassuring to rule out AI, especially in the absence of elevated cortisol-binding globulins [108].

Although laboratory testing is essential to confirm the diagnosis of adrenal insufficiency, both laboratory and patient errors can cause misleading results. One way to minimize these errors is to make certain that the different tests are internally consistent. Further complicating the diagnosis is the fact that the most common cause of primary adrenal insufficiency, autoimmune adrenalitis, is a process that usually worsens over a period of many months or years.

Morning Salivary Cortisol Concentration

A salivary cortisol concentration at 8 AM above 5.8 ng/mL (16 nmol/L) rules outAI, whereas a value below about 1.8 ng/mL (5 nmol/L) makes the presence of adrenal insufficiency likely.

Urinary Cortisol Measurements

Basal urinary cortisol excretion is low in patients with severe adrenal insufficiency, but may be low-normal in patients with partial adrenal insufficiency. Therefore, they cannot be used as a screening test for adrenal insufficiency.

Basal Plasma ACTH, Renin and Aldosterone Concentrations

Basal plasma ACTH concentration at 08:00h, when determined simultaneously with the measurement of basal serum cortisol concentration, would confirm the diagnosis of AI and establish the cause, however in most cases determination of ACTH is delayed. The normal values of basal 08:00h plasma ACTH concentrations range between 20-52 pg/mL (4.5-12 pmol/L). In primary AI, the 08:00h plasma ACTH concentration is elevated, and is coupled with increased concentration or activity of plasma renin, low aldosterone concentrations, hyperkalemia and hyponatremia. In secondary or tertiary AI, plasma ACTH and cortisol concentrations are low or low normal, associated with normal values of plasma concentrations of renin and aldosterone. In an acute setting (e.g., shock) it is crucial to determine if primary AI is the cause which can be confirmed by stimulating the adrenal gland with exogenous ACTH.

Short ACTH Stimulation Tests

A short ACTH stimulation test should be performed in all patients with a likely diagnosis of adrenal insufficiency, unless the diagnosis has been ruled out by a basal serum cortisol value in the upper end of the reference range or higher. The agent used is synthetic ACTH (1-24) (cosyntropin). In healthy individuals, cortisol responses are greatest in the morning, but in patients with adrenal insufficiency, the response to cosyntropin is the same in the morning and afternoon [111]. The Endocrine Society's 2016 Clinical Practice Guidelines suggest the 250 mcg standard high-dose test for most patients [112].

Standard High-Dose Test (250 mcg)

A normal response to the high-dose (250 mcg as an intravenous [IV] bolus)ACTH stimulation testis a rise in serum cortisol concentration after either 30 or 60 minutes to a peak of ≥18 to 20 mcg/dL (500 to 550 nmol/L) [113]. A normal response to the high-dose (250 mcg) ACTH stimulation test excludes primary adrenal insufficiency [114] and most patients with secondary adrenal insufficiency. In secondary AI of recent onset an insulin-induced hypoglycemia test or metyrapone test can confirm the diagnosis [108]. However, the high-dose test performs well when it is performed at least four months after surgery, or nine months after radiation therapy.

Low-Dose Test (1 mcg)

This test should be performed at 14:00h when the endogenous ACTH secretion is at its nadir [108]. The low-dose (1 mcg as an IV bolus) ACTH stimulation test criteria for a normal cortisol response after 20 or 30 minutes are variable: 17 to 22.5 mcg/dL (400 to 620 nmol/L) [115]. Because the 20-minute time point may provide the peak response in healthy individuals, it should be obtained routinely [116].The advantage of this test is that it can detect recent onset ACTH deficiency (secondary AI), partial AI and chronic partial AI that may be missed by the standard-dose test [108].

Prolonged ACTH Stimulation Tests

Prolonged stimulation with exogenous administration of ACTH helps differentiate between primary and secondary or tertiary AI. In secondary or tertiary AI, the adrenal glands respond with cortisol secretion following prolonged stimulation with ACTH, whereas in primary AI the adrenal glands are partially or completely destroyed and do not respond to ACTH. The prolonged ACTH test consists of the intravenous administration of 250 μg of ACTH as an infusion over eight hours (8-hour test) or over 24 hours on two (or three) consecutive days (two-day test), and the measurement of serum cortisol, and 24-hour urinary cortisol and 17-hydroxycorticoid (17-OHCS) concentrations before and after the infusion [108]. However this test is expensive, needs hospitalization and is rarely used. The low-dose ACTH test is recommended in suspicion of a new or recent onset ACTH deficiency (e.g., one to two weeks after pituitary surgery). High dose ACTH stimulation test is recommended for all other patients, including those who are more than four months post-pituitary surgery.

Adrenal Crisis

In an acutely ill patient with possible adrenal crisis, therapy should be initiated immediately with intravenous saline and glucocorticoids. The short ACTH stimulation test can be performed after initiation of glucocorticoid treatment provided that glucocorticoid therapy is not continued for more than a few days to avoid suppression of the HPA axis and impairment of the adrenal response [117].

Basal Plasma ACTH, Renin, and Aldosterone Concentration

When coupled with simultaneous measurement of basal serum cortisol, measurement of plasma ACTH may both confirm the diagnosis of adrenal insufficiency and establish its cause.

While a basal plasma ACTH, renin, and aldosterone measurement may be ordered with the cortisol measurement, treatment must proceed immediately without waiting for the test results. Often resuscitation includes empirichydrocortisone treatment so that the short ACTH stimulation test cannot be performed immediately.

- In primary adrenal insufficiency, the 8 AM plasma ACTH concentration is high, sometimes as high as or higher than 4000 pg/mL (880 pmol/L); these patients have mineralocorticoid deficiency in addition to cortisol deficiency, plasma renin concentration or activity will be elevated, while aldosterone levels will be low, with increased serum potassium and decreased serum sodium levels.
- In contrast, plasma ACTH concentrations are low or low normal in secondary or tertiary adrenal insufficiency. The normal value at 8 AM is usually between 20 and 52 pg/mL (4.5 and 12 pmol/L) in a

two-site chemiluminescent assay. Plasma levels of renin and aldosterone are usually unaffected in secondary or tertiary adrenal insufficiency, but mineralocorticoid deficiency can sometimes occur after very prolonged deficiency of ACTH. Serum sodium is often decreased with normal serum potassium secondary to increased vasopressin levels resulting from its decreased inhibition by cortisol.

Because glucocorticoid treatment can suppress ACTH secretion, blood samples for ACTH determination must be drawn before initiating glucocorticoid therapy or, in patients already being treated, at least 24 hours after the last dose of a short-acting glucocorticoid such ashydrocortisone and even longer after long-acting glucocorticoids such asdexamethasone. If the patient has been on replacement long-acting glucocorticoid therapy, the steroid should be replaced with hydrocortisone for several days before measuring the morning plasma ACTH.

Metyrapone Tests

Themetyrapone tests may be useful in occasional patients in whom partial ACTH deficiency is suspected, particularly in postoperative pituitary surgery patients and others with partial secondary adrenal insufficiency. Metyrapone blocks the final step in cortisol biosynthesis, resulting in reductions in cortisol secretion and the serum cortisol concentration, and stimulation of ACTH secretion in response to the decrease in cortisol negative feedback inhibition.

Insulin-Induced Hypoglycemia Test

This demands supervision while performing and it should be cautiously used only in patients with suspected recent ACTH deficiency or suspected growth hormone and ACTH deficiency. Insulin (usually at a dose of 0.15 units/kg; in patients with low basal cortisol levels, the dose should be reduced to 0.1 units/kg) is given to induce hypoglycemia of 35 mg/dL (1.9 mmol/L) or less. Cortisol concentrations are measured at 0, 30, and 45 minutes, even if glucose has been given to reduce symptoms of hypoglycemia.

Corticotropin-Releasing Hormone Test

It may be used to distinguish secondary from tertiary AI but from a therapeutic standpoint this distinction is rarely important. There is little or no ACTH response in patients with secondary or pituitary-related adrenal insufficiency, whereas patients with tertiary disease due to lack of CRH from the hypothalamus usually have an exaggerated and prolonged ACTH response [108]. As for now there are no optimal test protocol and criteria for interpretation of the test.

Autoantibody Screen

Adrenocortical antibodies or antibodies against 21-hydroxylase can be detected in more than 90% of patients with recent onset autoimmune adrenalitis [108].

Imaging

Patients without any associated autoimmune disease and negative autoantibody screen should undergo an adrenal CT. In cases of tuberculous adrenalitis, the CT scan shows initially hyperplasia of the adrenal glands with focal calcifications late during the course of the disease. Bilateral adrenal lymphoma, adrenal metastases or adrenal infiltration (sarcoidosis, amyloidosis, and hemochromatosis) may also be detected by CT scan. If central AI is suspected, a MR scan of the hypothalamus and pituitary gland should be performed. This may detect any potential CNS tumors [118].

Among all tests, the short high dose ACTH test is probably the single best (and simplest) test for confirming a diagnosis of chronic secondary AI [119]. The short low dose ACTH test or the metyrapone test may be substituted if new or recent onset ACTH deficiency is suspected.

The presence of X-linked adrenoleukodystrophy and adrenomyeloneuropathy should be excluded in young men, particularly in boys less than 15 years of age, who have idiopathic adrenal insufficiency without accompanying neurologic symptoms. It is estimated that approximately 8 percent of patients with this disorder have only adrenal involvement, while others may have early or preclinical disease when adrenal insufficiency is diagnosed.

Treatment of Chronic Adrenal Insufficiency

Patients should be informed that therapy will be life-long with dose adjustments according to the needs in stress periods. Patients should wear bracelets that provide information about their medical condition in emergencies. Patients should also have supplies of dexamethasone sodium phosphate and should be educated about how and when to administer them. Patients with AI should be treated with short-acting glucocorticoid hydrocortisone (10-12 mg/m2 body surface area) [120]. Glucocorticoid replacement should be monitored clinically, evaluating weight gain/loss, arterial blood pressure, annualized growth velocity and presence of Cushing features [121]. During minor illness or surgical procedures, glucocorticoids should be given at a dosage up to three times the usual maintenance dosage for up to three days. During major illness or surgery, high doses of glucocorticoid analogues are required to avoid an adrenal crisis. A continuous infusion of 10 mg of hydrocortisone per hour or the equivalent amount of dexamethasone or prednisolone eliminates the possibility of glucocorticoid deficiency. This dose can be halved the second postoperative day, and the maintenance dose can be resumed at the third postoperative day.

Mineralocorticoid Replacement Therapy

Mineralocorticoid replacement therapy is required to prevent intravascular volume depletion, hyponatremia and hyperkalemia. For these purposes, fludrocortisone (0.05 - 0.2 mg daily) should be taken in the morning. The dose of fludrocortisone is titrated individually based on the findings of clinical examination (mainly the body weight and arterial blood pressure) and the levels of plasma renin activity. If hypertension develops during the course of fludrocortisones treatment angiotensin II receptor blockers, angiotensin-converting enzyme inhibitors, or dihydropyridine calcium blockers may be initiated while fludrocortisone therapy continues [121].

Androgen replacement in the form dehydroepiandrosterone (25-50mg/day) is recommended in adult patients (especially premenopausal women), adolescents and children with AI but the levels of DHEA should be monitored before such treatment [121].

Treatment of Adrenal Crisis

The aim of initial management is to treat hypotension, hyponatremia and hyperkalemia, and to reverse glucocorticoid deficiency. Treatment should be started with immediate administration of i.v.100 mg hydrocortisone and rapid rehydration with normal saline infusion under continuous cardiac monitoring, followed by 100–200 mg hydrocortisone in glucose 5% per 24-hour continuous IV infusion. Once the patient's condition is stable and the diagnosis has been confirmed, parenteral glucocorticoid therapy should be tapered over 3-4 days and converted to an oral maintenance dose [120].

Treatment of Chronic Secondary and Tertiary AI

Glucocorticoid replacement is the mainstay similar to that in primary AI. Mineralocorticoid replacement is rarely required.

AI in Critically Ill Patients

Clinical manifestations of adrenal insufficiency are common in critically ill patients, specifically in patients with severe pneumonia, adult respiratory distress syndrome, sepsis, trauma, HIV infection, however absolute AI is rare [122]. Laboratory diagnosis of AI in crucially ill, especially in septic shock is not reliable. Hydrocortisone (<400 mg per day in divided doses) in septic shock with the addition of fludrocortisone (50 mcg via gastric tube once daily) is recommended. This combination is administered for 5 -7 days, and is tapered to withdrawal that is guided by the clinical response [123].

AI during Pregnancy

Adrenal insufficiency is relatively rare in pregnancy. Symptoms are usually “nonspecific,” such as nausea, vomiting and fatigue, making the diagnosis of adrenal insufficiency challenging. The current diagnostic tests are serum cortisol concentrations and the cosyntropin stimulation test [121].Peak cortisol response following ACTH stimulation is higher in pregnant than in non-pregnant women during the second and third trimesters, as a result of physiologic pregnancy-associated hypercortisolism and elevations of cortisol-binding globulin [108].

Regarding glucocorticoid replacement during pregnancy, hydrocortisone, cortisone acetate, prednisolone or prednisone can be administered; in contrast, fluorinated glucocorticoids such as dexamethasone should be avoided because they cross the placenta at higher rates [121]. During labor adequate saline hydration and 25 mghydrocortisone should be administered intravenously (IV) every six hours. At the time of delivery hydrocortisone should be given IV in a dose of 100 mg every six hours or as a continuous infusion. After delivery, the dose can be tapered rapidly to maintenance within three days. The regulation of plasma volume during pregnancy is complex. Patients should be followed closely throughout pregnancy for electrolyte abnormalities and signs of volume depletion. Plasma renin activity may be used as an index of adequate fludrocortisones dose [108].

AI in Infancy and Childhood

For children with primary adrenal insufficiency that is not due to congenital adrenal hyperplasia (CAH), the starting oral dose of hydrocortisone in the range of 7 to 10 mg/m^2/day [107]. Infants usually require somewhat higher doses for adequate replacement however the dose is substantially higher in children with CAH. The dose should then be titrated to the individual patient's needs depending on the clinical response and growth.

The hydrocortisone daily dose should be adjusted according to the increasing body surface area of the growing child. Caution should be paid to decreased growth velocity, excessive weight gain or other clinical manifestations suggestive of iatrogenic Cushing syndrome.

Children with primary AI also require fludrocortisones 0.1 mg/day with no further adjustments necessary. During the first 6 months, infants require supplementation of sodium chloride at a dose of 1-2 g/day administered in multiple feedings [112,118].

Adrenal Surgery

Surgical adrenalectomy is performed for benign (hormonally active or nonfunctional) and malignant tumors. Adrenalectomy is a challenging procedure and should only be performed by surgeons with specialized training. Adrenalectomy can be performed transabdominally, retroperitoneally, or transthoracically. The most common method is transabdominal adrenalectomy which can be conducted via an open or minimally invasive approach. Open transabdominal adrenalectomy can be performed via an anterior or thoracoabdominal approach while open retroperitoneal adrenalectomy is accomplished through a posterior approach. Minimally invasive approaches include laparoscopic transabdominal and posterior retroperitoneoscopic (RPA). Thoraco-abdominal adrenalectomy is used in the rare settings of very large tumors usually with diaphragmatic involvement or tumor extension into the chest.

Surgical Approach According to Adrenal Lesions

Adrenocortical Carcinoma (ACC)

In the United States, open adrenalectomy with removal of adjacent lymph nodes is recommended for known or suspected ACC, regardless of size. [124]. In Europe, laparoscopic adrenalectomy is performed for stage I or II ACC with a diameter <10 cm [125].

Pheochromocytoma

Adrenal pheochromocytomas can generally be removed laparoscopically when safe and feasible [126], conversion to open surgery in case of intraoperative bleeding (pheochromocytomas are hypervascular lesions) or capsular violation (risk of hypertensive crisis) [127]. Open adrenalectomy is recommended for large (>6 cm) or invasive pheochromocytomas [128], and for paragangliomas.

Adrenal Incidentaloma

Minimal invasive surgery (MIS) is the gold standard for removing benign adrenal masses, both functional and nonfunctional, including pheochromocytomas. MIS is preferred because of reduced blood loss, fewer intraoperative complications, earlier patient mobility, decreased length of stay, and faster return to regular activity compared with open surgery [129]. For large tumors (>10 cm) open surgery should be considered because of the malignant potential of the lesion, technical difficulties and complications if these lesions are approached with MIS.

Minimally invasive adrenalectomycan be performed with either the laparoscopic transabdominal or the posterior retroperitoneoscopic (RPA) approaches. MIS should not be performed in malignant tumor invasion.Laparoscopic transabdominal adrenalectomy is more widely adopted and is preferred for large tumors (>8 cm), obese patients, and when there is possibilityto convert to open surgery. RPA is preferred for patients with a history of extensive upper abdominal surgery and those who require bilateral adrenalectomies [130]. RPA can be safely performed for tumors ≤8 cm.

Bilateral Adrenalectomy

For patients with bilateral tumors or end-stage Cushing syndrome, RPA bilateral adrenalectomy is recommended.

Adrenal Metastasis

MIS adrenalectomy is the preferred approach for isolated adrenal metastasis from primary malignancies (e.g., lung cancer) when surgical resection is indicated [129]. In invasive lesions open adrenalectomy should be considered.

Retroperitoneoscopic Adrenalectomy

For patients who require bilateral adrenalectomies for benign tumors or isolated metastases, and who are not candidates for a transabdominal laparoscopic procedure, retroperitoneoscopic adrenalectomy (RPA) can be performed [131]. RPA is technically demanding and requires specific training and expertise.

Open Transabdominal Adrenalectomy

An open transabdominal adrenalectomy is typically performed in the following clinical settings to avoid rupture and spillage of malignant or large tumors [132]:

- Overt or suspected primary adrenal malignancy of any size (e.g., adrenal cortical carcinoma, malignant pheochromocytoma).
- Adrenal mass invading surrounding structures (e.g., liver, kidney, inferior vena cava).
- Bilateral benign adrenal masses not accessible to the laparoscopic approach.
- Extensive prior upper abdominal or retroperitoneal procedures that make a minimally invasive surgical (MIS) approach impossible.
- Concomitant procedures (e.g., hepatic resection) not amenable to laparoscopic approach.

Novel Techniques

As surgeon experience grows, evolving minimally invasive technologies such as robotic-assisted adrenalectomy and single-access retroperitoneoscopic adrenalectomy (SARA) are being developed. However, such procedures should only be performed in highly specialized centers by experienced care teams.

Robotic-Assisted Adrenalectomy

Robot-assisted techniques have been applied to both transabdominal and retroperitoneal adrenalectomy [133]. Retroperitoneal adrenalectomy particularly lends itself to a robot-assisted technique because the retroperitoneal space is limited and frequently requires dissection using angled instruments. A robot-assisted approach may be very useful in the retroperitoneoscopic approach for patients with a hostile abdomen or those requiring concomitant bilateral adrenalectomy, such as those with severe Cushing syndrome.

Numerous meta-analysis studies have compared outcomes between robotic-assisted and laparoscopic adrenalectomy with very few clear advantages for either approach, although robotic adrenalectomy was associated with a lower estimated blood loss, shorter hospital stay and longer operative time [134,135]. In another systemic review, RPA (retroperitoneal adrenalectomy) was more effective than LTA (transabdominal adrenalectomy) in terms of shorter operative time and hospital stay [136].

Single-Access Retroperitoneoscopic Adrenalectomy

The single-access retroperitoneoscopic adrenalectomy (SARA), a highly specialized procedure requiring specific expertise, has been shown to be safe and effective for patients with benign adrenal masses [137].

Partial Adrenalectomy

Partial adrenalectomy may be a reasonable alternative to complete adrenalectomy for small (<3cm), potentially benign adrenal lesions and may be preferred for bilateral small lesions [138]. Partial adrenalectomy has been reported with the laparoscopic transabdominal approach and the retroperitoneoscopic approach [138].

Postoperative Management

The length of stay is typically one to two days after an uncomplicated laparoscopic or retroperitoneoscopic adrenalectomy, while a hospitalization of three to five days is expected for patients undergoing an open adrenalectomy. Patient-controlled analgesia combined with the use of orally administered narcotics is the standard protocol for postoperative pain control.

Mortality and Mortality

Both open and [MIS] procedures are associated with a very low risk of mortality and morbidity rates range from 6 to 30 percent [139].MIS adrenalectomy is safe, effective, and less expensive than open adrenalectomy for patients with benign functional and nonfunctional adrenal masses. Studies reported that patients undergoing laparoscopic adrenalectomy had fewer postoperative complications than patients undergoing open adrenalectomy (10 versus 27 percent) [140] while intraoperative complication rates did not differ between the two groups.

Conclusion

The adrenal is a vital organ and dysfunction of the steroidogenic pathways for either glucocorticoid and mineralocorticoid synthesis can result in significant morbidity and mortality. The two very different parts of these glands, the medulla and cortex, regulate and maintain many of the body's internal processes—from metabolism to the fight-or-flight response. Identification of the endocrine dysfunction and initiation of appropriate treatment is essential for survival. Adrenal tumors can be identified by imaging, and adrenalectomy may be curative in experienced hands.

REFERENCES

[1] Kim S, Cho J (2017) *Oncologic imaging: urology.* Springer. https://doi.org/10. 1007/978-3-662-45218-9.

[2] Cerny JC (1977) Anatomy of the adrenal gland. *Urol Clin North Am* Jun 4(2): 169–177.

[3] Ishimoto H, Jaffe RB. Development and function of the human fetal adrenal cortex: a key component in the feto-placental unit. *Endocr. Rev.*2011 Jun; 32(3):317-55.

[4] Miller WL. The Hypothalamic-Pituitary-Adrenal Axis: A Brief History. *Horm Res Paediatr.*2018; 89(4):212-223].

[5] Burford NG, Webster NA, Cruz-Topete D. Hypothalamic-Pituitary-Adrenal Axis Modulation of Glucocorticoids in the Cardiovascular System. *Int J Mol Sci.*2017 Oct 16; 18(10).

[6] Megha R, Leslie SW. StatPearls [Internet]. StatPearls Publishing; Treasure Island (FL): Nov 13, 2018. *Anatomy, Abdomen and Pelvis, Adrenal Glands (Suprarenal Glands).*

[7] Baranowski ES, Arlt W, Idkowiak J. Monogenic Disorders of Adrenal Steroidogenesis. *Horm Res Paediatr.*2018; 89(5):292-310.

[8] Kline GA, Prebtani APH, Leung AA, Schiffrin EL. Primary aldosteronism: a common cause of resistant hypertension. *CMAJ.* 2017 Jun 05;189(22):E773-E778.

[9] Vaidya A, Dluhy R. Hyperaldosteronism. In: Feingold KR, Anawalt B, Boyce A, Chrousos G, Dungan K, Grossman A, Hershman JM, Kaltsas G, Koch C, Kopp P, Korbonits M, McLachlan R, Morley JE, New M, Perreault L, Purnell J, Rebar R, Singer F, Trence DL, Vinik A, Wilson DP, editors. *Endotext* [Internet]. MDText.com, Inc.; South Dartmouth (MA): Oct 19, 2016.

[10] Utriainen P, Laakso S, Liimatta J, Jääskeläinen J, Voutilainen R. Premature adrenarche--a common condition with variable presentation. *Horm Res Paediatr.*2015;83(4):221-31.

[11] Gounden V, Rampursat YD, Jialal I. Secretory tumors of the pituitary gland: a clinical biochemistry perspective. *Clin. Chem. Lab. Med.* 2018 Dec 19;57(2):150-164.

[12] Pourian M, Mostafazadeh DB, Soltani A. Does this patient have pheochromocytoma? A systematic review of clinical signs and symptoms. *J Diabetes Metab Disord.*2015;15:11.

[13] Paravati S, Warrington SJ. StatPearls [Internet]. StatPearls Publishing; Treasure Island (FL): Oct 27, 2018. *Physiology, Catecholamines.*

[14] Mattsson C, Young WF Jr. Primary aldosteronism: diagnostic and treatment strategies. *Nat Clin Pract Nephrol* 2006; 2:198.

[15] Roy S., Roy S. J., Pinard S., Agulleiro M. J., Cerdá-Reverter J. M., Parent J. L., and Gallo-Payet N. (2012)The C-terminal domains of melanocortin-2 receptor (MC2R) accessory proteins (MRAP1) influence their localization and ACTH-induced cAMP production. *Gen. Comp. Endocrinol.* 176, 265–274 [PubMed.

[16] Sundeep Malik, Terrance M. Dolan, Zachary J. Maben, and Patricia M. Hinkle; Adrenocorticotropic Hormone (ACTH) Responses Require Actions of the Melanocortin-2 Receptor Accessory Protein on the Extracellular Surface of the Plasma Membrane; *J Biol Chem.* 2015 Nov 13; 290(46): 27972–27985. doi:10.1074/jbc.M115. 668491.

[17] Smith SM, Vale WW. The role of the hypothalamic-pituitary-adrenal axis in neuroendocrine responses to stress. *Dialogues Clin Neurosci.* 2006;8(4):383-95. Review.

[18] Habib KE., Gold PW., Chrousos GP. Neuroendocrinology of stress. *Endocrinol Metab Clin North Am.* 2001;30:695–728.

[19] Vale W., Spiess J., Rivier C., Rivier J. Characterization of a 41 - residue ovine hypothalamic peptide that stimulates secretion of corticotropin and betaendorphin.*Science.*1981;213:1394–1397.

[20] Bamberger CM, Schulte HM., Chrousos GP. Molecular determinants of glucocorticoid receptor function and tissue sensitivity to glucocorticoids. *Endocr Rev.*1996;17:245–261.

[21] Yasir M, Kasi A. StatPearls [Internet]. StatPearls Publishing; Treasure Island (FL): Oct 27, 2018. *Multiple Endocrine Neoplasias, Type 2 (MEN II, Pheochromocytoma and Amyloid Producing Medullary Thyroid Carcinoma, Sipple Syndrome*).

[22] Wagner CA. Effect of mineralocorticoids on acid-base balance. *Nephron Physiol.*2014;128(1-2):26-.

[23] Bale TL., Vale WW. CRF and CRF receptors: role in stress responsivity and other behaviors. *Annu Rev Pharmacol Toxicol.* 2004;44:525–557.

[24] Dautzenberg FM., Hauger RL. The CRF peptide family and their receptors: yet more partners discovered. *Trends Pharmacol Sci.* 2002;23:71–77.

[25] Westphal NJ., Seasholtz AF. CRH-BP: the regulation and function of a phylogenetically conserved binding protein. *Front Biosci.* 2006;11:1878–1891.

[26] Antoni FA. Vasopressinergic control of pituitary adrenocorticotropin secretion comes of age. *Front Neuroendocrinol.* 1993;14:76–122.

[27] Hernando F., Schoots O., Lolait SJ., Burbach JP. Immunohistochemical localization of the vasopressin V1 b receptor in the rat brain and pituitary gland: anatomical support for its involvement in the central effects of vasopressin. *Endocrinology.* 2001;142:1659–1668.

[28] Raffin-Sanson ML., de Keyzer Y., Bertagna X. Proopiomelanocortin, a polypeptide precursor with multiple functions: from physiology to pathological conditions. *Eur J Endocrinol.* 2003;149:79–90.

[29] Cone RD., Lu D., Koppula S., et al. The melanocortin receptors: agonists, antagonists, and the hormonal control of pigmentation. *Recent Prog Horm Res.* 1996;51:287–317; discussion 318.

[30] Reul JM., de Kloet ER. Anatomical resolution of two types of corticosterone receptor sites in rat brain with in vitro autoradiography and computerized image analysis. *J Steroid Biochem.* 1986;24:269–272.

[31] McEwen BS. The neurobiology of stress: from serendipity to clinical relevance. *Brain Res.* 2000;886:172–189.[PubMed][Google Scholar].

[32] Herman JP., Figueiredo H., Mueller NK., et al. Central mechanisms of stress integration: hierarchical circuitry controlling hypothalamo-pituitary adrenocortical responsiveness. *Front Neuroendocrinol.* 2003;24:151–180.

[33] Plotsky PM., Cunningham ET., Jr Widmaier EP. Catecholaminergic modulation of corticotropin-releasing factor and adrenocorticotropin secretion. *Endocr Rev.* 1989;10:437–458.

[34] Kinzig KP., D'Alessïo DA., Herman JP., et al. CNS glucagon-like peptide-1 receptors mediate endocrine and anxiety responses to interoceptive and psychogenic stressors. *J Neurosci.* 2003;23:6163–6170.

[35] Johnson AK., Cunningham JT., Thunhorst RL. Integrative role of the lamina terminalis in the regulation of cardiovascular and body fluid homeostasis. *Clin Exp Pharmacol Physiol.* 1996;23:183–191.

[36] Aguilera G., Young WS., Kiss A., Bathia A. Direct regulation of hypothalamic corticotropin-releasing-hormone neurons by angiotensin II. *Neuroendocrinology.* 1995;61:437–444.[PubMed] [Google Scholar].

[37] Engelmann M., Landgraf R., Wotjak CT. The hypothalamic-neurohypophysial system regulates the hypothalamic-pituitary-adrenal axis under stress: an old concept revisited. *Front Neuroendocrinol.* 2004;25:132–149.

[38] Cullinan WE., Helmreich DL., Watson SJ. Fos expression in forebrain afférents to the hypothalamic paraventricular nucleus following swim stress. *J Comp Neurol.* 1996;368:88–99. [PubMed] [Google Scholar].

[39] Greco B., Allegretto EA., Tetel MJ., Blaustein JD. Coexpression of ER beta with ER alpha and progestin receptor proteins in the female rat forebrain: effects of estradiol treatment. *Endocrinology.* 2001;142:5172–5181.

[40] Raison CL., Miller AH. When not enough is too much: the role of insufficient glucocorticoid signaling in the pathophysiology of stress-related disorders. *Am J Psychiatry.* 2003;160:1554–1565.

[41] Forray Ml., Gysling K. Role of noradrenergic projections to the bed nucleus of the stria terminalis in the regulation of the hypothalamic-pituitary-adrenal axis. *Brain Res Brain Res Rev.* 2004;47:145–160.

[42] Herman JP., Mueller NK., Figueiredo H. Role of GABA and glutamate circuitry in hypothalamo-pituitary-adrenocortical stress integration. *Ann NY Acad Sci.* 2004;1018:35–45.

[43] Van de Kar LD., Blair ML. Forebrain pathways mediating stress-induced hormone secretion. *Front Neuroendocrinol.* 1999;20:1–48.

[44] Mayo-Smith WW, Song JH, Boland GL, et al. (2017) Management of incidental adrenal masses: a White Paper of the ACR Incidental Findings Committee. *J Am Coll Radiol.* https://doi.org/10.1016/j.jacr.2017.05.001.

[45] Johnson PT, Horton KM, Fishman EK (2009) Adrenal mass imaging with multidetector CT: pathologic conditions, pearls, and pitfalls. *Radiographics.* https://doi.org/10.1148/rg.295095027.

[46] Adam SZ, Nikolaidis P, Horowitz JM et al. (2016) Chemical shift MR imaging of the adrenal gland: principles, pitfalls, and applications. *Radiographics.* https://doi.org/10.1148/rg.2016150139.

[47] Chong S, Lee KS, Kim HY (2006) Integrated PET-CT for the characterization of adrenal gland lesions in cancer patients: diagnostic efficacy and interpretation pitfalls. *Radiographics.* https://doi.org/10.1148/rg.266065057.

[48] Elsayes KM, Mukundan G, Narra VR et al. (2004) Adrenal masses: MR imaging features with pathologic correlation. *Radiographics.* https://doi.org/10.1148/ rg.24si045514.

[49] Domenico Albano, Francesco Agnello, Federico Midiri et al, Imaging features of adrenal masses. *Insights into Imaging* (2019) 10:1 https://doi.org/10.1186/s13244-019-0688-8.

[50] Caoili E, Korobkin M, Francis IR et al. (2002) Adrenal masses: characterization with combined unenhanced and delayed enhanced CT. *Radiology.* https:// doi.org/10.1148/radiol.2223010766.

[51] Mayo-Smith WW, Boland GW, Noto RB et al. (2001) State-of-the-art adrenal imaging. *Radiographics.* https://doi.org/10.1148/radiographics.21.4. g01jl21995.

[52] Helck A, Hummel N, Meinel FG, Johnson T, Nikolaou K, Graser A (2014) Can single-phase dual-energy CT reliably identify adrenal adenomas? *Eur Radiol.* https://doi.org/10.1007/s00330-014-3192-z.

[53] Ho LM, Paulson EK, Brady MJ, Wong TZ, Schindera ST (2008) Lipid-poor adenoma on unenhanced CT: does histogram analysis increase sensitivity compared with a mean attenuation threshold? *AJR Am J Roentgenol.* https://doi.org/10.2214/AJR.07.3150.

[54] Rao P, Kenney PJ, Wagner BJ, Davidson AJ (1997) Imaging and pathologic features of myelolipoma. *Radiographics.* https://doi.org/10.1148/radiographics.17.6.9397452.

[55] Göran Åkerström, Genetic Syndromes Associated with Adrenal Tumors, Springer, *Adrenal glands* pp 251-264.

[56] Patel J, Davenport MS, Cohan RH, Caoili EM (2013) Can established CT attenuation and washout criteria for adrenal adenoma accurately exclude pheochromocytoma? *AJR Am J Roentgenol.* https://doi.org/10.2214/AJR.12.9620.

[57] Amodru V, Guerin C, Delcourt S et al. (2018) Quantitative (18)F-DOPA PET/CT in pheochromocytoma: the relationship between tumor secretion and its biochemical phenotype. *Eur J Nucl Med Mol Imaging.* https://doi.org/10. 1007/s00259-017-3833-y.

[58] Huang YC, Tang YL, Zhang XM, Zeng NL, Li R, Chen TW (2015) Evaluation of primary adrenal insufficiency secondary to tuberculous adrenalitis with computed tomography and magnetic resonance imaging: current status. *World J Radiol.* https://doi.org/10.4329/wjr.v7.i10.336.

[59] Jordan E, Poder L, Courtier J et-al (2012) Imaging of nontraumatic adrenal hemorrhage. *AJR Am J Roentgenol.* doi:https://doi.org/10.2214/AJR.11.7973.

[60] Sung YM, Lee KS, Kim BT et al. (2008) (18) F-FDG PET versus (18)F-FDG PET/CT for adrenal gland lesion characterization: a comparison of diagnostic efficacy in lung cancer patients. *Korean J Radiol.* https://doi.org/10.3348/kjr.2008.9.1.19.

[61] Galia M, Albano D, Picone D et al. (2018) Imaging features of pancreatic metastases: a comparison with pancreatic ductal adenocarcinoma. *Clin Imaging.*

[62] Wu Q, Luo W, Zhao Y, Xu F, Zhou Q (2017) The utility of 18F-FDG PET/CT for the diagnosis of adrenal metastasis in lung cancer: a PRISMA-compliant meta-analysis. *Nucl Med Commun.*

[63] Lonergan GJ, Schwab CM, Suarez ES et al. (2002) Neuroblastoma, ganglioneuroblastoma, and ganglioneuroma: radiologic-pathologic correlatıon. *Radiographics.*

[64] Leite NP, Kased N, Hanna RF et al. (2007) Cross-sectional imaging of extranodal involvement in abdominopelvic lymphoproliferative malignancies. *Radiographics.*https://doi.org/10.1148/rg.276065170.

[65] Ferrozzi F, Bova D (1995) CT and MR demonstration of fat within an adrenal cortical carcinoma. *Abdom Imaging* 20(3):272–274.

[66] Lynnette K. Nieman. *Recent Updates on the Diagnosis and Management of Cushing's Syndrome.*

[67] Kidambi S, Raff H, Findling JW. Limitations of nocturnal salivary cortisol and urine free cortisol in the diagnosis of mild Cushing's syndrome. *Eur J Endocrinol* 2007; 157:725.

[68] Alexandraki KI, Kaltsas GA, Isidori AM, Akker SA, Drake WM, Chew SL, et al. The prevalence and characteristic features of cyclicity and variability in Cushing's disease. *Eur J Endocrinol* 2009; 160:1011-8.

[69] Nieman LK, Biller BM, Findling JW, Murad MH, Newell-Price J, Savage MO, et al. Treatment of Cushing's syndrome: an Endocrine Society Clinical Practice Guideline. *J Clin Endocrinol Metab* 2015;100:2807-31.

[70] Lacroix A, Feelders RA, Stratakis CA, Nieman LK. Cushing's syndrome. *Lancet* 2015; 386:913-27.

[71] Fleseriu M, Biller BM, Findling JW, Molitch ME, Schteingart DE, Gross C, et al. Mifepristone, a glucocorticoid receptor antagonist, produces clinical and metabolic benefits in patients with Cushing's syndrome. *J Clin Endocrinol Metab* 2012; 97:2039-49.

[72] Lee F. Starker, John W. Kunstma, Tobias Carling. *Subclinical Cushing Syndrome: A Review.*

[73] Zeiger MA, Thompson GB, Duh QY, et al. American Association of Clinical Endocrinologists and American Association of Endocrine Surgeons Medical Guidelines for the Management of Adrenal Incidentalomas: executive summary of recommendations. *Endocr Pract* 2009; 15(5):450–3.

[74] Nieman LK, Biller BM, Findling JW, et al. The diagnosis of Cushing's syndrome: an Endocrine Society Clinical Practice Guideline. *J Clin Endocrinol Metab* 2008; 93(5):1526–40.

[75] Raff H, Findling JW. A physiologic approach to diagnosis of the Cushing syndrome. *Ann Intern Med* 2003; 138(12):980–91.

[76] Mantero F, Arnaldi G. Management approaches to adrenal incidentalomas. A view from Ancona, Italy. *Endocrinol Metab Clin North Am* 2000; 29(1): 107–25, ix.

[77] Chiodini I, Morelli V, Masserini B, et al. Bone mineral density, prevalence of vertebral fractures, and bone quality in patients with adrenal incidentalomas with and without subclinical hypercortisolism: an Italian multicenter study. *J Clin Endocrinol Metab* 2009; 94(9):3207–14.

[78] Barzon L, Fallo F, Sonino N, et al. Development of overt Cushing's syndrome in patients with adrenal incidentaloma. *Eur J Endocrinol* 2002; 146(1):61–6.

[79] Rossi R, Tauchmanova L, Luciano A, et al. Subclinical Cushing's syndrome in patients with adrenal incidentaloma: clinical and biochemical features. *J Clin Endocrinol Metab* 2000; 85(4):1440–8.

[80] Speiser PW. *Congenital Adrenal Hyperplasia.* F1000Res. 2015 Aug 20;4(F1000 Faculty Rev):601. doi: 10.12688/f1000research.6543.1. Collection 2015. Review.

[81] Auchus RJ, Arlt W: Approach to the patient: the adult with congenital adrenal hyperplasia. *J Clin Endocrinol Metab.* 2013; 98(7): 2645–55.

[82] New MI, Tong YK, Yuen T, et al.: Noninvasive prenatal diagnosis of congenital adrenal hyperplasia using cell-free fetal DNA in maternal plasma. *J Clin Endocrinol Metab.* 2014; 99(6): E1022–30.

[83] Falhammar H, Frisén L, Norrby C, et al.: Increased mortality in patients with congenital adrenal hyperplasia due to 21-hydroxylase deficiency. *J Clin Endocrinol Metab.* 2014; 99(12): E2715–21.

[84] Quinkler M, Stewart PM. Hypertension and the cortisol-cortisone shuttle. *J Clin Endocrinol Metab* 2003; 88:2384.

[85] Adamidis A, Cantas-Orsdemir S, Tsirka A, et al. Apparent Mineralocorticoid Excess in the Pediatric Population: Report of a Novel Pathogenic Variant of the 11β-HSD2 Gene and Systematic Review of the Literature. *Pediatr Endocrinol Rev* 2019; 16:335.

[86] Stewart PM. Tissue-specific Cushing's syndrome, 11beta-hydroxysteroid dehydrogenases and the redefinition of corticosteroid hormone action. *Eur J Endocrinol* 2003; 149:163.

[87] Ulick S, Wang JZ, Blumenfeld JD, Pickering TG. Cortisol inactivation overload: a mechanism of mineralocorticoid hypertension in the ectopic adrenocorticotropin syndrome. *J Clin Endocrinol Metab* 1992; 74:963.

[88] Dave-Sharma S, Wilson RC, Harbison MD, et al. Examination of genotype and phenotype relationships in 14 patients with apparent mineralocorticoid excess. *J Clin Endocrinol Metab* 1998; 83:2244.

[89] Palermo M, Delitala G, Mantero F, et al. Congenital deficiency of 11beta-hydroxysteroid dehydrogenase (apparent mineralocorticoid excess syndrome): diagnostic value of urinary free cortisol and cortisone. *J Endocrinol Invest* 2001; 24:17.

[90] Palermo M, Shackleton CH, Mantero F, Stewart PM. Urinary free cortisone and the assessment of 11 beta-hydroxysteroid dehydrogenase activity in man. *Clin Endocrinol (*Oxf) 1996; 45:605.

[91] Farese RV Jr, Biglieri EG, Shackleton CH, et al. Licorice-induced hypermineralocorticoidism. *N Engl J Med* 1991; 325:1223.

[92] Käyser SC, Dekkers T, Groenewoud HJ, et al. Study Heterogeneity and Estimation of Prevalence of Primary Aldosteronism: A

Systematic Review and Meta-Regression Analysis. *J Clin Endocrinol Metab* 2016; 101:2826.
[93] Mattsson C, Young WF Jr. Primary aldosteronism: diagnostic and treatment strategies. *Nat Clin Pract Nephrol* 2006; 2:198.
[94] Monticone S, D'Ascenzo F, Moretti C, et al. Cardiovascular events and target organ damage in primary aldosteronism compared with essential hypertension: a systematic review and meta-analysis. *Lancet Diabetes Endocrinol* 2018; 6:41.
[95] Funder JW, Carey RM, Mantero F, et al. The Management of Primary Aldosteronism: Case Detection, Diagnosis, and Treatment: An Endocrine Society Clinical Practice Guideline. *J Clin Endocrinol Metab* 2016; 101:1889.
[96] Weinberger MH, Fineberg NS. The diagnosis of primary aldosteronism and separation of two major subtypes. *Arch Intern Med* 1993; 153:2125.
[97] Young WF. Primary aldosteronism: renaissance of a syndrome. *Clin Endocrinol* (Oxf) 2007; 66:607.
[98] Prada ETA, Burrello J, Reincke M, Williams TA. Old and New Concepts in the Molecular Pathogenesis of Primary Aldosteronism. *Hypertension* 2017; 70:875.
[99] Funder JW, Carey RM, Fardella C, et al. Case detection, diagnosis, and treatment of patients with primary aldosteronism: an endocrine society clinical practice guideline. *J Clin Endocrinol Metab* 2008; 93:3266.
[100] Harper R, Ferrett CG, McKnight JA, et al. Accuracy of CT scanning and adrenal vein sampling in the pre-operative localization of aldosterone-secreting adrenal adenomas. *QJM* 1999; 92:643.
[101] Rossi GP, Auchus RJ, Brown M, et al. An expert consensus statement on use of adrenal vein sampling for the subtyping of primary aldosteronism. *Hypertension* 2014; 63:151.
[102] Lim V, Guo Q, Grant CS, et al. Accuracy of adrenal imaging and adrenal venous sampling in predicting surgical cure of primary aldosteronism. *J Clin Endocrinol Metab* 2014; 99:2712.

[103] Young WF, Stanson AW, Thompson GB, et al. Role for adrenal venous sampling in primary aldosteronism. *Surgery* 2004; 136:1227.

[104] Monticone S, Auchus RJ, Rainey WE. Adrenal disorders in pregnancy. *Nat Rev Endocrinol* 2012; 8:668.

[105] Kong MF, Jeffocoate W. Eighty-six cases of Addison's disease. *Clin Endocrinol* (Oxf) 1994; 41(6):757-61.

[106] Claire Burton, Addison's disease: identification and management in primary care, *Br J Gen Pract.* 2015 Sep; 65(638): 488–490. doi:10.3399/bjgp15X686713.

[107] Neary N, Nieman L. Adrenal insufficiency: etiology, diagnosis and treatment. *Curr Opin Endocrinol Diabetes Obes* 2010; 17(3):217-23.

[108] NicolaidesNC, Chrousos GP, Charmandari E. *Adrenal Insufficiency. Endotext* [Internet]. South Dartmouth (MA): MDText.com, Inc.; 2000-.2017 Oct 14 PMID: 25905309.

[109] Oelkers W. Adrenal insufficiency. *N Engl J Med* 1996; 335:1206.

[110] Hägg E, Asplund K, Lithner F. Value of basal plasma cortisol assays in the assessment of pituitary-adrenal insufficiency. *Clin Endocrinol* 1987; 26:221.

[111] Burgos N, Ghayee HK, Singh-Ospina N. Pitfalls in the interpretation of the cosyntropin stimulation test for the diagnosis of adrenal insufficiency. *Curr Opin Endocrinol Diabetes Obes* 2019; 26:139.

[112] Bornstein SR, Allolio B, Arlt W, et al. Diagnosis and Treatment of Primary Adrenal Insufficiency: An Endocrine Society Clinical Practice Guideline. *J Clin Endocrinol Metab* 2016; 101:364.

[113] Thaler LM, Blevins LS Jr. The low dose (1-microg) adrenocorticotropin stimulation test in the evaluation of patients with suspected central adrenal insufficiency. *J Clin Endocrinol Metab* 1998; 83:2726.

[114] Oelkers W, Diederich S, Bähr V. Diagnosis and therapy surveillance in Addison's disease: rapid adrenocorticotropin (ACTH) test and measurement of plasma ACTH, renin activity, and aldosterone. *JClin Endocrinol Metab* 1992; 75:259.

[115] Rasmuson S, Olsson T, Hagg E. A low dose ACTH test to assess the function of the hypothalamic-pituitary-adrenal axis. *Clin Endocrinol* (Oxf) 1996; 44:151.

[116] Park YJ, Park KS, Kim JH, et al. Reproducibility of the cortisol response to stimulation with the low dose (1 microg) of ACTH. *Clin Endocrinol* (Oxf) 1999; 51:153.

[117] Broide J, Soferman R, Kivity S, et al. Low-dose adrenocorticotropin test reveals impaired adrenal function in patients taking inhaled corticosteroids. *J Clin Endocrinol Metab* 1995; 80:1243.

[118] Boland GW. Adrenal imaging: from Addison to algorithms. *Radiol Clin North Am* 2011; 49(3):511-28.

[119] Streeten DH. What test for hypothalamic-pituitary-adrenocortical insufficiency? *Lancet* 1999; 354:179.

[120] Falorni A, Minarelli V, Morelli S. Therapy of adrenal insufficiency: an update. *Endocrine* 2013; 43(3):514-28.

[121] Bornstein SR, Allolio B, Arlt W, Barthel A, Don-Wauchope A, Hammer GD, Husebye ES, Merke DP, Murad MH, Stratakis CA, Torpy DJ. Diagnosis and Treatment of Primary Adrenal Insufficiency: An Endocrine Society Clinical Practice Guideline. *J Clin Endocrinol Metab.* 2016; 101(2):364-89.

[122] Fleseriu M, Loriaux DL. "Relative" adrenal insufficiency in critical illness. *Endocr Pract* 2009; 15(6):632-40.

[123] Marik PE, Pastores SM, Annane D, Meduri GU, Sprung CL, Arlt W, Keh D, Briegel J, Beishuizen A, Dimopoulou I, Tsagarakis S, Singer M, Chrousos GP, Zaloga G, Bokhari F, Vogeser M; American College of Critical Care Medicine. Recommendations for the diagnosis and management of corticosteroid insufficiency in critically ill adult patients: consensus statements from an international task force by the American College of Critical Care Medicine.*Crit Care Med* 2008; 36(6):1937.

[124] Zeiger MA, Thompson GB, Duh QY, et al. American Association of Clinical Endocrinologists and American Association of Endocrine Surgeons Medical Guidelines for the Management of Adrenal

Incidentalomas: executive summary of recommendations. *Endocr Pract* 2009; 15:450.

[125] Gaujoux S, Mihai R, joint working group of ESES and ENSAT. European Society of Endocrine Surgeons (ESES) and European Network for the Study of Adrenal Tumours (ENSAT) recommendations for the surgical management of adrenocortical carcinoma. *Br J Surg* 2017; 104:358.

[126] https://www.nccn.org/professionals/physician_gls/pdf/neuroendocrine.pdf (Accessed on May 31, 2017).

[127] Taffurelli G, Ricci C, Casadei R, et al. Open adrenalectomy in the era of laparoscopic surgery: a review. *Updates Surg* 2017; 69:135.

[128] Lenders JW, Duh QY, Eisenhofer G, et al. Pheochromocytoma and paraganglioma: an endocrine society clinical practice guideline. *JClin Endocrinol Metab* 2014; 99:1915.

[129] Carr AA, Wang TS. Minimally Invasive Adrenalectomy. *Surg Oncol Clin N Am* 2016; 25:139.

[130] Lombardi CP, Raffaelli M, De Crea C, et al. Endoscopic adrenalectomy: Is there an optimal operative approach? Results of a single-center case-control study. *Surgery* 2008; 144:1008.

[131] Callender GG, Kennamer DL, Grubbs EG, et al. Posterior retroperitoneoscopic adrenalectomy. *Adv Surg* 2009; 43:147.

[132] Mir MC, Klink JC, Guillotreau J, et al. Comparative outcomes of laparoscopic and open adrenalectomy for adrenocortical carcinoma: single, high-volume center experience. *Ann Surg Oncol* 2013; 20:1456.

[133] Taskin HE, Berber E. Robotic adrenalectomy. *Cancer J* 2013; 19:162.

[134] Economopoulos KP, Mylonas KS, Stamou AA, et al. Laparoscopic versus robotic adrenalectomy: A comprehensive meta-analysis. *Int J Surg* 2017; 38:95.

[135] Brandao LF, Autorino R, Laydner H, et al. Robotic versus laparoscopic adrenalectomy: a systematic review and meta-analysis. *Eur Urol* 2014; 65:1154.
[136] Chai YJ, Kwon H, Yu HW, et al. Systematic Review of Surgical Approaches for Adrenal Tumors: Lateral Transperitoneal versus Posterior Retroperitoneal and Laparoscopic versus Robotic Adrenalectomy. *Int J Endocrinol* 2014; 2014:918346.
[137] Dickson PV, Jimenez C, Chisholm GB, et al. Posterior retroperitoneoscopic adrenalectomy: a contemporary American experience. *J Am Coll Surg* 2011; 212:659.
[138] Miron A, Giulea C, Nădrăgea M, et al. Laparoscopic Partial Adrenalectomy. *Chirurgia* (Bucur) 2017; 112:77.
[139] Walz MK, Groeben H, Alesina PF. Single-access retroperitoneoscopic adrenalectomy (SARA) versus conventional retroperitoneoscopic adrenalectomy (CORA): a case-control study. *World J Surg* 2010; 34:1386.
[140] Gill IS. The case for laparoscopic adrenalectomy. *J Urol* 2001; 166:429.

BIOGRAPHICAL SKETCH

Levent Soydan

Affiliation: Department of Radiology, Haydarpasa Numune Education and Research Hospital, Istanbul, Turkey

Education: Radiologist, MD

Research and Professional Experience: Practising radiologist for 22 years

Professional Appointments: Sifa Hospital, Medamerican Hospital Istanbul

Publications from the last 3 years:

1) Soydan L, Eren Ozturk H, Onal ZE, Nuhoglu C. Associations ofthyroid volume and function with childhood obesity. *Acta Endocrinol* (Buchar). 2019 Jan-Mar;-5(1):123-128. doi: 10.4183/ aeb.2019.123.
2) Soydan L, Demir AA, Ozer S, Ozkara S. Can MR Enterography and Diffusion-Weighted Imaging Predict Disease Activity Assessed by Simple Endoscopic Score for Crohn's Disease? *J Belg Soc Radiol.* 2019 Jan 18;103(1):10. doi: 10.5334/jbsr.1521.
3) Karaca H, Soydan L, Yildiz S, Toros SZ. Measurement of the depth of facial nerve at the level of stylomastoid foramen using MR imaging in Bell's palsy. *Clin Imaging.* 2019 Nov-Dec;58:34-38. doi: 10.1016/ j.clinimag.2019.06.008. Epub 2019 Jun 14.
4) Soydan L, Gündoğdu H, Aslan A, Inan I, Balık AO. Bilateral inguinal hernia with an uncommon content: A case report. *Acta Gastroenterol Belg.* 2016 Sep-Dec;79(3):495-496.
5) Önal ZE,Soydan L, Öztürk HE, Sağ Ç, Gürbüz T, Nuhoğlu Ç, Şimşek MM.Carotid intima media thickness in obese children: is there an association with hyperlipidemia? *J Pediatr Endocrinol Metab.* 2016 Feb;29(2):157-62. doi: 10.1515/jpem-2015-0221.
6) Soydan L, Demir AA, Sayman E, Onomay Celik B, Oven Ustaalioglu BB.Adrenal mass of unusual etiology: Ewing sarcoma in a young man. *Radiol Case Rep.* 2017 Jul 31;12(4):838-844. doi: 10.1016/ j.radcr. 2017.07.002. eCollection 2017 Dec.
7) Onal ZE,Soydan L, Karadas B, Gurbuz T, Nuhoglu C, Simsek MM. Management of chronic cervical lymphadenopathy in a group of children. *Minerva Pediatr.* 2016 Feb 19.
8) Soydan L, Demir AA, Tunaci A. Frequency of abnormal pulmonary computed tomography findings in asylum seeking refugees in Turkey. *Int Health.* 2017 Mar 1;9(2):118-123. doi: 10.1093/inthealth/ihw057.

In: The Pituitary Gland and Adrenal Glands ISBN: 978-1-53617-605-6
Editor: Noémi Barta

Chapter 6

GLUCOCORTICOID-INDUCED ADRENAL INSUFFICIENCY: POTENTIAL RISK PREDICTORS AND DIAGNOSIS

*A. B. Mañas-Martínez**, PhD*
and M. Mañas-Martínez
Department of Diabetes and Endocrinology,
Ernest Lluch Hospital, Calatayud, Spain
Deparment of Internal Medicine, Clinico Hospital, Zaragoza, Spain

ABSTRACT

Glucocorticoids are widely used for the treatment of various inflammatory conditions, malignancies and after organ transplantation. The use of glucocorticoids is associated with numerous side effects. Glucocorticoids are considered the most common cause of tertiary adrenal insufficiency. Therefore, patients may require glucocorticoid replacement therapy after chronic use of glucocorticoids.

There are few studies in the published literature that have approached the assessment of the hypothalamo-pituitary-adrenal axis function

* Corresponding Author's E-mail: anab.manas@gmail.com.

following glucocorticoid therapy. As a result, there has been little consensus in the components of glucocorticoid exposure (dose and time) that may contribute to the hypothalamo-pituitary-adrenal axis suppression and potential recovery. The general approach in most centers is to gradually taper the dose of glucocorticoids to diminish the risk of adrenal insufficiency following glucocorticoid withdrawal.

This paper is aimed to obtain knowledge about the risk of developing adrenal insufficiency among glucocorticoid users and identify risk factors. Secondary aims are to explore if some features of the hypothalamo-pituitary-adrenal axis function testing could guide physicians to identify those groups of patients at higher risk of presenting with adrenal insufficiency.

Keywords: glucocorticoid, withdrawal, adrenal insufficiency, short synacthen test, basal cortisol

INTRODUCTION

Glucocorticoids (GCs) are widely used for the treatment of various conditions, such as inflammatory and rheumatologic diseases. GCs have established as the main immunosuppressive therapy alongside standard immunosuppressant drugs after organ transplantation. In general, the prevalence of population taking chronic glucocorticoid (GC) therapy has been estimated at 0.9% in the UK [1]. Among most common indications for oral long-term GC treatment were inflammatory arthropathies (19.3%) and respiratory diseases (6.1%) [1].

Despite their anti-inflammatory and immunosuppressive effects, GCs are well - known for their important side effects such as hypertension, proximal myopathy, osteoporosis, diabetes mellitus and depression. Tertiary adrenal insufficiency (AI) is one of the most feared complications among treating physicians [2]. Nowadays GC therapy is the most common cause of suppression of the hypothalamic-pituitary-adrenal (HPA) axis. GC -induced AI results from negative feedback of exogenous GCs in the pituitary and hypothalamus glands, which interferes with secretion of corticotropin- releasing hormone (CRH) and adrenocorticotropic hormone (ACTH). As a consequence endogenous cortisol production is reduced and is insufficient during acute conditions such as infection, surgery and major trauma [3]. The EU-AIRE study reported a mortality of 1,5% for patients with GC -induced AI presenting with an adrenal crisis [3]. Therefore, it is vital to detect AI among GC users and provide them with adequate GC replacement therapy, especially under acute circumstances [4].

FREQUENCY OF HYPOTHALAMIC-PITUITARY-ADRENAL SUPPRESSION AND GLUCOCORTICOID THERAPY

GC -induced AI is probably underestimated in clinical practice. A recent retrospective, record- linkage study in primary and hospital care in England has shown a frequency of 0.3% over 450,816 person-years of follow-up. The low observed absolute risk of GC -induced AI is probably secondary to the presence of low reports of the problem. This is likely due to the lack of awareness of GC -induced AI among physicians, with few GC users being diagnosed with the condition [5].

The dominating clinical focus has been on AI following withdrawal of GCs. Tapering GC regimen is commonly used in an attempt to reduce the probability of GC -induced AI [6]. Not only AI can be observed after GC withdrawal but also during ongoing low-dose prednisolone treatment. GC - induced AI has been observed in more than one-third of patients with rheumatoid arthritis and in 43% renal transplant patients on 5 or 7.5 mg of prednisolone daily administered for a period of at least 6 months [7, 8]. The daily dose, the duration and the cumulative dose of GC therapy are correlated with the degree of HPA axis function in treated patients [9]. There is substantial evidence of GC -induced AI following low dose and short- term therapy of GCs. Adrenal failure has been observed early after initiation of GC treatment [10-12]. In general, there is a correlation between the dosage and duration of therapy and GC -induced AI. Nevertheless, this correlation is little and there is not any threshold either in time or dose that can predict GC -induced AI [9]. Furthermore, there is interindividual variability response to GC therapy and HPA axis suppression. In a pharmacogenomic assessment performed in a cohort of asthma and chronic obstructive respiratory disease patients, it was observed that common variants in the *PDGFD* gene (e.g., rs591118) were associated with the development of GC -induced AI [13].

PREDICTING THE HYPOTHALAMIC-PITUITARY-ADRENAL AXIS SUPPRESSION

GC -induced HPA axis suppression shows an individual pattern. GCs can cause complete central suppression of ACTH with adrenal gland atrophy. The suppression can be partial, being adrenal gland only not able to meet the additional requirements of cortisol during acute conditions. In some patients suppression of the HPA axis may not exist at all [6].

The suppression of the HPA axis is associated with the potency of the specific GC drug. It is related to the half-life of the drug and the duration of ACTH suppression [6]. Hydrocortisone and cortisone acetate are the least potent and suppressive agents. Prednisone, prednisolone, methylprednisolone and triamcinolone are moderate potent GCs. Dexamethasone is the GC with the longest biological half- life and therefore suppress ACTH in the most intensive manner.

When GCs are given at a frequency that does not allow the HPA axis to recover between doses, patients are at higher risk for HPA axis suppression [14].

Administration form of GC is related to the HPA axis suppression. Oral and intra-articular administration is associated with AI in around half of the patients [15]. In patients taking inhaled GCs without receiving additional systemic therapy, GC -induced AI can be present in 7.8% and up to 20% of the patients [15, 16]. The HPA axis suppression is less frequent with topical administration (4.7%) [15]. It can be observed after 1-2 weeks of initiating treatment. Nevertheless, adrenal recovery is fast and cortisol levels return to normal levels within few weeks despite continuous therapy [15]. Patients with chronic inflammatory skin disease with impaired barrier function who require prolonged GC treatment can be on special danger of GC -induced AI. There have been some reports of AI associated with topical GC, when they have been administered in either higher doses or longer than maximum recommended. The side effects of topical GCs should always be kept in mind, especially when dealing with patients with chronic inflammatory skin disease [18].

The time of the day of delivery of GC has been associated with the suppression of the HPA axis [6]. Midnight administration of GC suppresses cortisol secretion from the adrenal gland in a very intensive manner. Multiple daily dose administration is not secure and assures suppression of the HPA axis. A single morning dose regimen shows potency in controlling symptoms with less side effects, being the recommended regimen [19].

The daily and cumulative dose of GCs and the duration of the treatment are correlated with the degree of the HPA axis suppression [6, 10-12, 14-16]. In a prospective study of 9 patients hospitalized for acute exacerbation of chronic obstructive pulmonary disease, 78% had a blunted peak cortisol response on the first day of administration of GCs [11]. The HPA axis suppression persisted for a variable period of time after a standardized steroid treatment consisting in a single injection of 40 mg of methylprednisolone followed by an oral 13-day regime of 40 mg prednisone). Furthermore, 33% of the patients maintained suppressed their HPA axis on day 14 after GC cessation [11]. After a single epidural GC injection, cortisol production can be diminished for even a period of 14 days [10]. In a systematic review and meta-analysis of the percentage of patients with AI following GC withdrawal, use of GCs in low, medium or high doses resulted in a percentage of AI of 2.4%, 8.5% and 21.5%, respectively [15]. Use of GCs for a short, medium, or long-term resulted in a percentage of AI of 1.4%, 11.9%, and 27.4%, respectively [15]. Recovery of the HPA axis suppression was associated with the dose and duration of GCs [15]. 38.7% of the patients presented with GC -induced AI after 4 weeks of short-term and high-dose GC treatment. 61.4% of them recovered few weeks after and had their HPA axis intact. On the other hand, long-term and medium-dose GC therapy was associated with more frequency of AI after 6 months of GC withdrawal (56.4%). Half of them (25.3%) remained with GC -induced AI 6 months after [15]. Another systematic review of 73 studies retesting patients after GC withdrawal found evidence of persisting GC -induced AI, ranged from 75% (after 10 weeks of cessation) to 15% (after 3 years of cessation) [12]. The groups of patients analyzed were exposed to different dose and duration of GC therapy. There was no obvious pattern when stratifying by the dose, duration or cumulative dose. However, there was an association between the median cumulative dose of GC received and persisting AI. The median percentage of patients with GC -induced AI ranged from 14% for a medium cumulative dose (0.5–5 g) to 50% for a high cumulative dose (greater than 5 g) [12].

Basal cortisol level on the patient that is still on treatment can be helpful to diagnose AI [20]. In a retrospective study of 404 patients on long-term GC treatment, an ambulatory morning cortisol of 410 nmol/l (15 mcg/dl) had 100% specificity for predicting passing the Short Synacthen Test (SST) and a serum cortisol of 34 nmol/l (1.23 mcg/dl) was 99% sensitive for predicting AI [16].

Common symptoms of AI such as weakness, low blood pressure and hypoglycemia are very unspecific and do not help to identify the patient at risk of having AI. Hyponatremia and adrenal crises can present in only 18% of patients [22]. In general, clinical signs and symptoms of AI are not unable to predict an impairment of the HPA-axis. This should be kept in mind before AI is discarded in the patient on GCs without "typical" clinical symptoms and signs of AI.

To conclude, it could be said that there are some predictors of GC -induced AI such as the potency of the administered GC, the cumulative dose and the duration of GC treatment. Basal cortisol level of the patient on GCs can help to detect the patient that is likely to suffer from AI. Nevertheless, in every individual patient is not possible to completely exclude the presence of GC -induced AI.

ASSESSMENT OF ADRENAL INSUFFICIENCY BEFORE GLUCOCORTICOID WITHDRAWAL

The diagnosis of AI is biochemical. The gold-standard test to detect the HPA axis recovery is the Insulin Tolerance Test (ITT). This test uses a small bolus dose of insulin to induce hypoglycemia. Cortisol is then measured before the bolus and over 120 min after the bolus [2, 6, 21]. The criteria for a normal serum cortisol response ranges from 500 to approximately 600 nmol/l (18-22 mcg/dl), depending on the reference of the laboratory assay [22]. The ITT is cumbersome to perform. Moreover, this test is contraindicated in patients with coronary heart disease, cerebrovascular disease or epilepsy [2].

The SST is the most widely used test in the initial assessment of AI [2, 6, 21, 22]. A standard high -dose and a low- dose SST are available. Low-dose test is no more effective than high- dose test in detecting AI. Thus, the standard high- dose SST is the preferred dynamic test in clinical practice [2, 6, 21, 22]. In the high -dose SST, 0.25 mg of ACTH [1-24] is administered intravenously or intramuscular. Cortisol is measured at 0,30 and 60 min after. In healthy individuals, cortisol response is greatest in the morning but in patients with AI the response to ACTH is the same in the morning and afternoon [20]. It is always best to perform the test in the morning to avoid a false negative result in a healthy subject. In clinical practice, patients who achieve a peak cortisol concentration of 500–600 nmol/l (18-22 mcg/dl) at 30–60 min following ACTH are usually defined as having normal adrenal reserve [2, 6, 21, 22].

In practice, the SST and ITT correlate well. Assuming the IST as the gold standard, the sensitivity of SST to detect adrenal failure is between 70% and 85% with specificity between 82% and 96% [24]. During the SST a 30 min plasma cortisol value of 600 nmol/l is more reliable than a value of 500 nmol/l, and using the former criterion the SST can safely be used as a first line test for the evaluation of the HPA axis. However, if the result is borderline or there is clinical suspicion of mild hypocorticotrophism an ITT should be warranted [25]. ITT remains the best test to establish the presence of adrenal failure when clinical suspicion persists in a patient with a "normal" SST [20].

The results generated from the SST can provide useful information to predict the likelihood of the HPA axis recovery [26]. In a retrospective analysis of SST performed in 110 patients with current or previous GC exposure, the incremental response of cortisol in the SST was predictor of future recovery of the HPA axis. 95% of patients who had an initial incremental response >100 nmol/l (3.6 mcg/dl) showed a normal cortisol response in the SST within a 4-year follow-up. In the group with an incremental response <100 nmol/l, 67% recovered. The combination of the incremental response to SST and a basal cortisol differentiated better the patients that would recover from GC-induced adrenal suppression. An incremental cortisol <100 nmol/l (3.6 mcg/dl) with a basal cortisol of >200 nmol/l (7.3 mcg/dl) predicted a shorter median time to recovery (322 days; CI 95%: 134-357). A basal cortisol <200 nmol/l (7.3 mcg/dl) predicted little chance of recovery in at least a 4-year period [26].

Morning serum cortisol level is safe and easy to perform and is a good initial assessment of adrenal function. It helps to determine the need for dynamic tests like the SST, which are more expensive and time-consuming [27]. Morning serum cortisol can show variability as total cortisol concentrations depend on corticosteroid-binding globulin (CBG) and albumin concentrations. Increased CBG is associated with estrogen use and during pregnancy [2, 21, 28]. For this reason, it is advisable to discontinue estrogen therapy for a period of at least six weeks prior to determining basal cortisol [22]. During pregnancy it should be used a higher cortisol cut-off to diagnose adrenal failure [28, 29]. Reduction of production of CBG can be seen in hepatic failure, hypothyroidism and sepsis. Nephrotic syndrome is associated with renal losses of CBG [2, 28]. These conditions may lead to misleadingly diminished total serum cortisol concentrations despite normal biologically active free cortisol [28]. Furthermore, there exists inter- assay variability and cortisol cut-off should be determined depending on the assay method used in local practice [22].

Cortisol levels are usually undertaken between 7:00-9:00 am, at the time of maximum peak of cortisol and in the absence of replacement therapy (at least 18 hours after the last dose of GC). Intact HPA axis is determined with a basal morning cortisol of more than 500 nmol/l (18 mcg/dl) [21]. According to guidelines, patients with levels of <100 nmol/l (3.6 mcg/dl) are diagnosed straightaway of AI and are advised to commence with GC replacement and stress supplementation if needed [2, 21, 28]. In the intermediate range, basal levels >365 nmol/l (13 mcg/dl) can predict AI with a positive predictive value of 91% [28].

There are some studies that have analyzed the level of basal cortisol that can accurately predict AI in the patient on GC therapy [16, 20, 27, 30]. In a study of 404 patients exposed to different forms of GC therapy, a serum cortisol concentration of 34 nmol/l (1.23 mcg/dl) was 100% sensitive for predicting failure [16]. The same cut-off was determined in patients on inhaled GC therapy [16]. A retrospective study conducted in 505 patients to determine the predictive value of morning serum cortisol in determining an adequate response in the SST, a basal morning cortisol of >375 nmol/l (13.6 mcg/dl) had a specificity of 95% and a positive predictive value of 95% to determine adrenal sufficiency, although its sensitivity to exclude AI was only 43% [27]. A cortisol level >236 nmol/l (8.5 mcg/dl) showed better sensitivity (84%) at the expense of less specificity (71%) [27]. Baseline cortisol ≥223.5 nmol/l (8 mcg/ dl) had a specificity of 100% for passing the SST and a sensitivity of 72.73% in 27 patients with glomerular disease on chronic GC treatment [30]. A similar cut-off (242 nmol/l (8.8 mcg/dl) has shown as predictor of adequate SST in a retrospective review of 33 patients diagnosed with AI after a median 2-year period of GC treatment. Its sensitivity was similar (70%) but showing better specificity (93%) [20]. A higher cortisol cut-off (410 nmol/l (15 mcg/dl)) had the highest specificity (100%) for predicting normal adrenal response to SST [16]. A basal cortisol cut-off of <100 nmol/l has shown specificity of 100% in predicting adrenal failure [27].

ACTH level remains either low or normal after GC therapy. It does not help in the diagnosis of GC-induced AI [32].

It can be standard practice to screen patients on chronic GC treatment with an ambulatory morning cortisol on a regular basis during follow-up. On this way, an adequate assessment of the adrenal reserve will perform

[20]. A basal cortisol of 100 nmol/l (3.6 mcg/dl) is straightly linked to GC-induced AI and determines the initiation of GC replacement therapy. It could be affirmed that a basal cortisol level >375 nmol/l (13.6 mcg/dl) is highly predictive of a normal response of the HPA axis, not requiring dynamic testing to assess the HPA axis. A morning cortisol even higher (410 nmol/l (15 mcg/dl)) predicts normal adrenal response to SST with a specificity of 100% [16]. A cortisol level in an undetermined range (100 (3.6 mcg/dl) and 375 (13.6 mcg/dl) nmol/l) would determine the need of performing a SST to evaluate the HPA axis [16]. In the case of a cortisol between 236 and 375 nmol/l (8.5- 13.6 mcg/dl), morning cortisol level could be reassessed and SST considered if clinical suspicion persist [20].

This testing strategy can be applied in clinical practice with the majority of patients with suspected GC-induced AI correctly diagnosed. Nevertheless, it should keep in mind that clinical assessment should be above biochemical testing. Strong clinical suspicion of GC-induced AI should be confirmed with SST regardless of the basal cortisol level. ITT remains the best test that completely excludes GC-induced AI when cortisol levels after SST are within the normal range [25].

WITHDRAWING GLUCOCORTICOID THERAPY

Attempts are made to make GC therapy safer. To prevent or minimize side effects secondary to GC therapy, GC tapering to the lowest dose necessary to maintain control of disease activity is recommended. GC tapering also permits the recovery of the HPA axis suppression [31, 32].

It is important to consider factors that make more likely the presence of AI in the patient taking GCs. GC dose and duration of therapy is associated with GC- induced AI [15]. Although there is no administration form, dose or treatment duration for which the risk of AI can be safely excluded. The general approach is to estimate the patient as high risk of AI if 5-7.5 mg of prednisone has been administered for more than 3 weeks [31, 33]. The patient on low and medium GC dose for more than a year is in special risk of AI [15]. In these groups of patients is especially important to taper patients off GCs.

The guidance of GC tapering regimes given in the literature is not based on controlled clinical trials [6, 12, 34, 35]. Studies with different GC tapering schemes in rheumatoid arthritis did not include objective outcome variables to evaluate the efficacy and success of the schemes. A systematic review found insufficient evidence about the efficacy in controlling the disease and safety of different GC tapering regimens [34]. Studies comparing GC tapering regimens are needed [33, 34].

Once the disease is stable, an approach is reducing the GC dose 10-20 percent every 2-4 weeks and monitor the clinical response of the patient [33]. Once a patient´s dosage has been tapered to a prednisone dosage of 5 mg per day and if the disease is quiescent, many physicians could opt to continuing to taper the dosage until the GC is completely withdrawn [6]. The physician will need to follow the patient and test for AI in the case symptoms or signs of AI appear.

Another approach is to exclude the presence of AI with the performance of SST once the patient is on a stable physiological GC dose [6, 16, 20]. An alternative is to perform a morning cortisol after at least 18 hours of the last GC dose [16, 20]. This can reduce the number of dynamic tests performed, as cortisol levels can evaluate the adrenal reserve. The interpretation of cortisol level could be done according the proposed algorithm described in the above section. To summarize, if cortisol is >375 nmol/l (13.6 mcg/dl), this is highly predictive of a normal HPA axis response and the patient does not require SST. A basal cortisol of 100 nmol/l (3.6 mcg/dl) is diagnostic of AI and the patient should be converted to hydrocortisone replacement and should be instructed in self-administration of supplemental hydrocortisone during acute stress. Parenteral hydrocortisone should be administered during severe stress and in patients who cannot take medicines by mouth. Patients should undergo SST if morning cortisol is in the indeterminate range. SST will determine if the patient can be successfully be tapered of GCs.

Conclusion

GCs are commonly used to control a broad spectrum of diseases. Their use can produce side effects such as obesity, diabetes, and osteoporosis. GC-induced AI is a potentially fatal complication. GC dose and duration of therapy is associated with AI. However, there is no defined lower limit dose and duration of therapy where zero risk of AI exists. GC- induced AI can occur while the patient is on chronic GC treatment and may persist several months after GC withdrawal. In the current review it has presented an approach to detect the patient at risk of presenting with GC-induced AI before GC withdrawal. This management is based on the morning cortisol and helps to identify the patient that can benefit from dynamic testing (SST).

References

[1] van Staa, T.P., Leufkens, H.G., Abenhaim, L., Begaud, B., Zhang, B. and Cooper, C. (2000). Use of oral corticosteroids in the United Kingdom. *QJM: montly journal of the Association of Physician*, 93(II): 105-111.

[2] Charmandari, E., Nicolaides, N.C. and Chrousos, G.P. (2014). Adrenal insufficiency. *Lancet*, 383: 2152–2167.

[3] Hahner, S., Loeffler, M., Bleicken, B., Drechsler, C., Milovanovic, D., Fassnacht, M., Ventz, M., Quinkler and M., Allolio, B. (2010). Epidemiology of adrenal crisis in chronic adrenal insufficiency: the need for new prevention strategies. *European journal of Endocrinology*, 162 (III): 597-602.

[4] Dineen, R., Thompson, C.J. and Sherlock, M. (2019). Adrenal crisis: prevention and management in adult patients. *Therapeutic advances in Endocrinology and Metabolism*, 10: 1-12.

[5] Teumzghi, F.M., Morgan, A.W., Keeley, A., Baxter, P.D., Stewart, P.M. and Pujades-Rodriguez, M. (2019). Dose dependency of

iatrogenic glucocorticoid excess and adrenal insufficiency and mortality: a cohort study in England. *The Journal of Clinical Endocrinology and Metabolism,* 104 (IX): 3757–3767.

[6] Krasner, A. (1999). Glucocorticoid-induced adrenal insufficiency. *Journal* of the American Medical Association, 282(VII): 671-676.

[7] Borresen, S.W., Klose, M., Baslund, B., Rasmussen, A.K., Hilsted, L., Friis-Hansen, L., Locht, H., Hansen, A., Hetland, M.L., Lydolph, M.C. and Feldt- Rasmussen, U. (2017). Adrenal insufficiency is seen in more than one-third of patients during ongoing low-dose prednisolone treatment for rheumatoid arthritis. *European journal of Endocrinology*, 177(IV): 287-295.

[8] Valentin, A., Borresen, S.W., Rix, M., Elung-Jensen, T., Sorensen, S.S. and Feldt-Rasmussen, U. (2019). Adrenal insufficiency in kidney transplant patients during low-dose prednisolone therapy: a cross-sectional case-control study. *Nephrology, dialysis, transplantation.* doi: 10.1093/ndt/gfz180. [Epub ahead of print]

[9] Schlaghecke, R., Kornely, E., Santen, R.T. and Ridderskamp, P. (1992). The effect of long-term glucocorticoid therapy on pituitary adrenal responses to exogenous corticotropin-releasing hormone. *The New England Journal of Medicine*, 326 (IV): 226-230

[10] Abdul, A.J., Ghai, B., Bansal, D., Sachdeva, N., Bhansali, A. and Dhatt, S.S. (2017). Hypothalamic pituitary adrenocortical axis suppression following a single epidural injection of methyl-prednisolone acetate. *Pain Physician Journal,* 20(VII): 991- 1001.

[11] Schuetz, P, Christ-Crain, M., Schild, U., Süess, E., Facompre, M., Baty, F., Nusbaumer, C., Brustche, M., and Müller B. (2008). Effect of a 14-day course of systemic corticosteroids on the hypothalamic-pituitary-adrenal axis in patients with acute exacerbation of chronic obstructive pulmonary disease. *BMC pulmonary medicine,* 8:1.

[12] Joseph, R.M., Hunter, A.L., Ray, D.W. and Dixon, W.G. (2016). Systemic glucocorticoid therapy and adrenal insufficiency in adults: A systematic review. *Seminars in Arthritis and Rheumatism,* 46(I): 133-141.

[13] Hawcutt, D.B., Francis, B., Carr, D.F., Jorgenesen, A.L., Yin, P., Wallin, N., O´Hara, N., Zhang, E.J., Bloch, K.M., Ganguli, A., Thompson, B., McEvoy, L., Peak, M., Crawford, A.A., Walker, B.R., Blair, J.C., Couriel, J., Smyth, R.L. and Pirmohamed, M. (2018). Susceptibility to corticosteroid-induced adrenal suppression: a genome-wide association study. *The Lancet. Respiratory medicine*, 6(VI), 442- 450.

[14] Sacre, K., Dehoux, M., Chauveheid, M.P., Chauchard, M., Lidove, O., Roussel, R.,and Papo, T. (2013). Pituitary-Adrenal Function After Prolonged Glucocorticoid Therapy for Systemic Inflammatory Disorders: An Observational Study. *The Journal of Clinical Endocrinology and Metabolism*, 98(VIII): 3199–3205

[15] Broersen, L.H., Pereira, A.M., Jorgensen, J.O. and Dekkers, O.M. (2015). Adrenal Insufficiency in Corticosteroids Use: Systematic Review and Meta-Analysis. *The Journal of Clinical Endocrinology and Metabolism,* 100 (VI): 2171-2180.

[16] Woods, C.P., Argese, N., Chapman, M., Boot, C., Webster, R., Dabhi, V., Grossman, A.B., Toogood, A.A., Arlt, W., Stewart, P.M., Crowley, R.K. and Tomlinson, J.W. (2015). Adrenal suppression in patients taking inhaled glucocorticoids is highly prevalent and management can be guided by morning cortisol. *European Journal of Endocrinology*, 173(V): 633-642.

[17] Levin, E., Gupta, R., Butler, D., Chiang, C. and Koo, J.Y.M. (2014). Topical steroid risk analysis: Differentiating between physiologic and pathologic adrenal suppression. *The journal of Dermatological Treatment*, 25(VI): 501-506.

[18] Böckle, B.C., Jara, D., Nindl, W., Aberer, W. and Sepp, N.T. (2014). Adrenal insufficiency as a result of long-term misuse of topical corticosteroids. *Dermatology*, 228: 289-293.

[19] Alten, R. and Wiebe, E. (2015). Hypothalamic -Pituitary -Adrenal axis function in patients with rheumatoid arthritis treated with different glucocorticoid approaches. *Neuroimmunodulation*, 22: 83-88.

[20] Leong, S.H., Shander, S. and Ratnasingam, J. (2018). Predicting recovery of the hypothalamic-pituitary-adrenal axis after prolonged glucorticoid use. *Endocrine practice*, 24(I): 14-20.

[21] Grossman, A.B. (2010). The diagnosis and management of central hypoadrenalism. *The Journal Clinical Endocrinology and Metabolism,* 95 (XI): 4855- 4863.

[22] Wallace, I., Cunningham, S., and Lindsay, John. (2009). The diagnosis and investigation of adrenal insufficiency in adults. *Annals of Clinical Biochemistry*, 46: 351–367.

[23] Fleseriu, M., Gassner, M., Yedinak, C., Chicea, L., Delashaw, J.B. and Loriaux, D.L. (2010). Normal hypothalamic-pituitary-adrenal axis by high-dose cosyntropin testing in patients with abnormal response to low-dose cosyntropin stimulation: a retrospective review. *Endocrine Practice*, 16(I). 64-70.

[24] Giordano, R., Picu, A., Bonelli, L.L., Balbo, M., Berardelli, R., Marinazzo, E., Corneli, G., Ghigo, E. and Arvat, E. (2008). Hypothalamus-pituitary-adrenal axis evaluation in patients with hypothalamo-pituitary disorders: comparison of different provocative tests. *Clinical Endocrinology,* 68: 935-941.

[25] Bangar, V. and Clayton, R.N. (1998). How reliable is the short synacthen test for the investigation of the hypothalamic-pituitary-adrenal axis? *European Journal of Endocrinology,* 139(VI): 580-3.

[26] Pofi, R., Feliciano, C., Sbardella, E., Argese, N., Woods, C.P., Grossman, A.B., Jafar-Mohammadi, B., Gleeson, H., Lenzi, A., Isidori, A.M. and Tomlinson, J.W. (2018). The Short Synacthen (Corticotropin) Test can be used to predict recovery of hypothalamo-pituitary-adrenal axis function. *The Journal Clinical Endocrinology and Metabolism,* 103(VIII):3050-3059.

[27] Yo, W.S., Toh, L.M., Brown, S.J., Howe, W.D., Henley, D.E. and Lim, E.M. (2014). How good is a morning cortisol in predicting an adequate response to intramuscular synacthen stimulation? *Clinical Endocrinology*, 81(I): 19-24.

[28] De Miguel-Novoa, P., Vela, E.T., Rodríguez, N.M., Guerras, I.S., Martínez de Salinas-Santamaría, M.L. and Masó, A.A. (2014).

Guidelines for the diagnosis and treatment of adrenal insufficiency in the adult. *Endocrinologia y Nutrición*, 61 (SI): 1-35.

[29] Yuen KC, Chong LE and Koch CA. (2013). Adrenal insufficiency in pregnancy: challenging issues in diagnosis and management. *Endocrine,* 44:283-92.

[30] Karangizi, A.H.K., AI-Shaghana, M., Logan, S., Criseno, S., Webster, R., Boelaert, K., Hewins, P. and Harper, L. (2019). Glucocorticoid induced adrenal insufficiency is common in steroid treated glomerular diseases - proposed strategy for screening and management. *BMC Nephrology*, 20(I): 154.

[31] Guerrero-Pérez, F., Marengo, A.P. and Villabona-Artero, C. (2017). The unresolved riddle of glucocorticoid withdrawal. *Journal of Endocrinological Investigation,* 40, 1175-1181.

[32] Dinsen, S., Baslund, Bo., Klose, M., Rasmussen, A.K., Friis-Hansen, L., Hilsted, L. and Feldt-Rasmussen, U. (2013). Why glucocorticoid withdrawal may sometimes be as dangerous as the treatment itself. *European Journal of Internal medicine*, 24: 714-720.

[33] Furst, D., Saag, K. *Glucocorticoid withdrawal.* https://www-uptodate-com./contents/glucocorticoid-withdrawal. Accessed October 10, 2019.

[34] Volkmann, E.R., Rezai, S., Tarp, S., Woodworth, T.G. and Furst, D.E. (2013). We still don´t know how to taper glucocorticoids in rheumatoid arthritis, and we can do better. *Journal of Rheumatology*, 40 (X): 1646-1649.

[35] Ritcher, B., Neises, G. and Clar, C. (2002). Glucocorticoid withdrawal schemes in chronic medical disorders. A systematic review. *Endocrinology and Metabolism Clinics of North America,* 31 (III): 751-778.

In: The Pituitary Gland and Adrenal Glands
Editor: Noémi Barta
ISBN: 978-1-53617-605-6

Chapter 7

SIGNIFICANCE OF ADRENAL GLAND FOR HEAT STRESS AMELIORATION IN LIVESTOCK

***M. V. Silpa*[1], *J. P. Anisha*[2], *G. D. Vandana*[3], *S. P. Angel*[3], *M. R. Reshma Nair*[3,4] and *V. Sejian*[4,*]**

[1]Institute of Animal Breeding and Genetics, Justus-Liebig-University Gießen, Gießen, Germany
[2]Kerala Veterinary and Animal Sciences University, Mannuthy, Thrissur, Kerala
[3]Academy of Climate Change Education and Research, Kerala Agricultural University, Vellanikkara, Thrissur, Kerala, India
[4]ICAR-National Institute of Animal Nutrition and Physiology, Adugodi, Hosur Road, Bangalore

ABSTRACT

The rising global temperature has been a major concern in livestock production as it affects the productive performance of livestock across the

---

[*] Corresponding Author's E-mail: drsejian@gmail.com.

globe. Heat stress has been proven to be detrimental to the livestock industry and has resulted in huge economic losses due to reduction in production. Domestic animals exhibit various biological response mechanisms to survive the harsh climatic conditions and neuro-endocrine regulation of stress response was considered the primary mechanisms by which the animals survive the stress. The hypothalamic-pituitary-adrenal (HPA) axis activation is a potent and complex response to heat stress in domestic livestock. The HPA axis is activated during stress which leads to the secretion of cortisol and aldosterone, from adrenal gland. The cortisol secreted from adrenal cortex was considered to be the ideal stress marker in livestock. The cortisol which is the primary glucocorticoid released from the adrenal cortex, mainly target liver, muscle and adipose tissue to initiate gluconeogenesis, glycogenolysis, lipolysis and proteolysis mechanisms in stressed animals thereby restoring their energy homeostasis while aldosterone maintains the electrolyte balance in them. The release of these steroid hormones plays a vital role to ameliorate heat stress in farm animals. Being the prime sensor of stress, the adrenal gland plays a significant role in maintaining homeostasis and thereby reducing the detrimental effects of heat stress in livestock.

Keywords: adrenal gland, heat stress, cortisol, aldosterone, HPA axis

1. Introduction

Livestock production covers more than 45 per cent of the Earth's usable land surface, most of which are subjected to harsh and varying climatic conditions. These variations in environmental conditions are expected to have severe impacts on livestock production systems across the globe. Apart from hampering the economy and welfare of the animals, this would also affect the global food supply. The livestock sector plays a central role to cater the food demands of the exponentially rising population. Though the increasing demand for livestock products are offering improved market opportunities for the small scale, marginal and landless farmers, the changing climatic scenario is putting them under higher pressure as it affects the productivity of these animals (Sejian et al., 2015).

Predominantly the livestock sector is located in regions experiencing harsh environmental conditions thereby subjecting the animals to stress. Among all the stressors, heat stress is of prime concern as it has a devastating impact on the livestock industry. Heat stressed animals utilize most of their energy to maintain homeostasis as a result of which a reduction in their growth rate, reproductive efficiency, milk production and increased susceptibility to diseases may be observed. Apart from these direct consequences of heat stress, it also has an indirect effect on the animal's productivity by adversely affecting the water and pasture availability and reducing the yield of other fodder resources for the animals (Baumgard et al., 2012). All these factors converge down, causing a multifold deleterious impact on the livestock production thus causing huge economic losses to the farmers.

Animals adapt various strategies to combat the adverse effects of heat stress and neuro-endocrine responses play a key role in maintaining homeostasis in animals. The secretions of the adrenal gland which is activated by the hypothalamic-pituitary-adrenal axis (HPA) are the chief regulators of heat stress. Glucocorticoids and mineralocorticoids, secreted from the adrenal cortex, are the primary hormones, involved in alleviating heat stress in animals (Afsal et al., 2018). Glucocorticoids elicit physiological changes in animals thus aiding them to cope with the stress. They enhance hepatic gluconeogenesis and also act as a vasodilator to dissipate heat (Cunningham and Klein, 2007). Mineralocorticoids, predominantly aldosterone regulates the electrolyte and fluid homeostasis in heat stressed animals. Thus, the secretions from the adrenal gland play a vital role in amelioration of heat stress in animals.

The secretions from the adrenal gland are mediated via the HPA axis, which involves a complex set of direct and feedback interactions between the hypothalamus, pituitary and adrenal gland. For the prominent role it plays in stress relieving pathway, this axis is also called as stress axis. The axis follows a cascade of events primarily with the hypothalamus release of corticotrophin-releasing Factor (CRF) as a response to the stress signal by the animal. The CRF acts on the anterior pituitary gland leading to the release of adrenocorticotropic hormone (ACTH). It is the ACTH that finally binds to the receptors on the adrenal cortex, to stimulate the release of cortisol, the predominant glucocorticoid involved in heat stress assessment and alleviation (Binsiya et al., 2017). There are a number of factors influencing the activation of this axis and it is of prime importance to understand them thoroughly so as to ameliorate heat stress.

2. Heat Stress Impact on Livestock

Livestock production provides a sustainable source of income for a major proportion of marginal small scale farmers across the globe. It was estimated to contribute nearly 30 per cent to the world's Gross Domestic Products (GDP). However, with the changing climatic scenario, the livestock sector has been exposed to a number of threats (Pragna et al., 2017). Heat stress, one of the main environmental stress variables, has a direct and/or indirect impact on livestock industries. It affects livestock production, reproduction, animal's health status, fodder production and natural resources management.

The primary responses exhibited by animals to combat heat stress are increased respiration rate, body temperature, water consumption and reduction in feed intake. While increase in respiratory rate, body temperature and water consumption help to dissipate heat from the animal, reduction in feed intake prevents metabolic heat generation on digestion (Sejian et al., 2015). Apart from this, exposure of animals to heat stress may also lead to a significant reduction in feed conversion ratio. The decrease in anabolic activity and increase in tissue catabolism influence the growth and average daily weight gain in livestock.

Milk production is probably the most severely affected trait in dairy cattle as a consequence of thermal stress. High milk producing cattle are more affected due to their higher internal metabolic heat generation which makes them more vulnerable to heat stress. The feeding pattern, rumen functions and udder health of lactating animals are altered during heat stress thereby resulting in a reduction in milk production by the animal (Pragna et al., 2017). Heat stress also affects the milk quality leading to a reduction in milk fat, solids-not-fat, milk protein and lactose content. Additionally, lower levels of calcium, phosphorus and magnesium and high chloride values are observed in the milk of animals exposed to heat stress (Bernabucci et al. 2013).

During the harsh climatic conditions, heat stressed animals would have to walk longer distances in search of fodder and water. Depletion in both the quantity and quality of grazing land is a common phenomenon in the changing climate scenario thereby leading to undernourishment in animals. Exposure to thermal stress has been proven to influence reproductive processes in animals (Sejian et al., 2011). Heat stress has been proven to reduce the estradiol levels in animals. Glucocorticoids disrupt the reproductive cycle in animals by acting on the hormonal pathway involved in it. Glucocorticoids enhance the negative feedback of estradiol also in addition to reducing the stimulation of gonadotropin releasing hormone (GnRH) receptor expression by oestrogen (Sejian, 2013). This results in an increase in silent estrus, reduction in conception rate and also affects parturition in animals. Apart from influencing the reproductive cycle, thermal stress also influences embryo production (Naqvi et al., 2004). The birth weight of lambs born from heat stressed does were reported to be lower thereby indicating an impact of heat stress on foetal development (Sejian, 2013).

Global climate change causes a huge alteration in the ecological construction. These changes enhance the efficiency, transmission and widen the host spectrum of various pathogens and parasites thereby increasing the disease susceptibility of animals. Additionally, climate change and associated environmental stress affect the pasture and fodder availability to livestock (Sejian et al., 2015). The harsh climatic conditions would reduce the harvested forage yield and alter its nutritional value thereby depriving the animals from adequate nourishment. Lack of quality fodder and water would further hamper the productivity of the animals, the outcome of which would be huge economic losses to the farmers. Thus impact of climate change on livestock production is immense and proper ameliorative strategies should be adopted to reduce the stress on livestock.

3. Biological Mechanisms of Livestock to Cope with Heat Stress

The animals tend to alter several biological mechanisms to survive in extreme climatic conditions, the process known as adaptation mechanisms, which includes physiological, behavioural, blood biochemical and neuro-endocrine and cellular and molecular mechanisms.

The heat stressed animals exhibit several behavioral changes including reduction in feed intake, water drinking frequency, shade seeking behavior, lying and standing time, wallowing, urination and defecation.

During high temperature exposure, animals tend to reduce the feed intake as a part of adaptation in an effort to reduce metabolic heat production to cope with external hot environment. Increased drinking frequency is another behavioral adaptation in ruminants during high ambient temperature. Generally water consumption of livestock raises during increase in temperature by 20-30% and rise in every degree increases 0.81 L of water consumption (Athira et al., 2017). Sheeps in arid region tend to concentrate their urine so as to balance higher water loss (Gaughan et al., 2019). Shade seeking behavior is yet another behavioural adaptation seen in livestock during high temperature exposure. Heat stress also alters the standing and lying time in livestock. Change in the temperature leads to more standing time in cows so as to increase evaporative heat loss from the body and aid in convection. Heat stressed animals tend to stand more to reduce conductive and radiative heat from the ground which ultimately reduces their lying time. Wallowing is another behavioural adaptation seen in buffaloes and pigs. Wallowing enhances grazing time and production in buffalo heifers as it helps to maintain the body temperature during heat stress. Frequency of urination and defecation varies with changing environmental conditions and generally animals exposed to high ambient temperature shows reduced defecation and urination frequency (Athira et al., 2017).

Alteration in physiological variables such as respiration rate, pulse rate, skin and rectal temperature is one of the primary mechanisms by which the animals survive the heat stress. Infact respiration rate and rectal temperatures are established to be confirmatory physiological biomarker for heat stress in different livestock species. However, breed variations are established in physiological mechanisms and generally indigenous livestock species show much less variations in their physiological responses as compared to exotic animals which are susceptible to heat stress.

The blood biochemical composition significantly helps in assessing the health status of animals. Heat stress influences the blood biochemical constituents such as packed cell volume (PCV), hemoglobin (Hb), plasma glucose, albumin, total protein, total cholesterol, non-esterified fatty acid (NEFA) in animals. When animal is under heat stress they tend to increase hemoglobin and packed cell volume as a part of adaptation (Mazzullo et al., 2014). The reduced PCV during heat stress could be attributed to the excess requirement of water in the circulatory system in order to dissipate the heat through haemodilution effect (Garkal et al., 2016). In an effort to adapt heat stress, animals tend to decrease the secretion of thyroid hormones to control the metabolic activities in an effort to reduce body heat production. Further, heat stress raises the levels of blood cortisol and is considered an important biological marker for quantifying heat stress in livestock (Sejian et al., 2012). Blood glucose level also reduces in heat stressed animals as adaptation is biologically a costly process and it involves regular supply of glucose to maintain vital body functions. Generally, metabolic activities are maintained by the mobilization and utilization of non-esterified fatty acid (NEFA) during the stressful conditions. The plasma level of NEFA reduces as a result of long time exposure of the animal to heat stress. This is due to the high requirement of NEFA in the liver and peripheral tissues as a source of energy (Skibiel et al., 2018). The total serum cholesterol also shows a decreasing pattern in animals during high ambient temperatures.

Neuro- endocrine responses plays a major role in animal adaptation. Heat stress induces variation in the secretion of pituitary hormones, leading to changes in metabolism, immune competence and behaviour, as well as failures in reproduction (Binsiya et al., 2017). The hormones that are significant to heat stress adaptation includes glucocorticoids, catecholamines, antidiuretic hormone (ADH), thyroid hormones, mineralo-corticoids, growth hormone (GH) and prolactin (PRL). Increase in the environmental temperature activates the hypothalamic-pituitary adrenocortical axis (HPA) and sympatho–adrenal medullary axis (SAM). The HPA axis is involved in regulation of the stress response in livestock (Shaji et al., 2017). The HPA axis also maintains the production of glucocorticoids which act as the stress relieving hormone in heat stressed animals (Ribeiro et al., 2018). Further, the animals subjected to short term stress increases the production of plasma cortical while the production reduces during chronic stress. Another vital endocrine secretion from adrenal gland is the aldosterone which helps in regulation of electrolyte mechanism. When the animals are subjected to heat stress they are prone for dehydration which activates the renin-angiotensin-aldosterone pathway to reinstate fluid and electrolyte balance (Afsal et al., 2018).

4. Economic Consequences of HS on Livestock Production

The livestock sector is one of the fastest emerging dominant agricultural subsectors in the world and it plays a major role in global economy. Approximately 30% of the planet's ice-free terrestrial surface area is occupied by the livestock sector and it is serving as a major source of income for poor people and directly supports and sustains livelihood security of 766 million marginal farmers in the developing countries (Food and Agriculture Organization, FAO, 2015).

Further, livestock sector is a major component of the agriculture and it contributes around 36% of the global agricultural GDP, which is also projected to have an increase of 50-60% in the coming decades (Thornton, 2010). In India, livestock sector account for 40% of the national GDP (Sejian et al., 2016). Recent projections clearly showed that the global demand for livestock and its products may increase by around 70%, to meet the demand of rapidly growing human population which is projected to reach 9.6 billion by 2050 (FAO, 2015).

Increasing urbanization, population, and purchasing power increase the requirements of livestock products and they satisfy the nutritional demand of the world through high quality meat and milk. The livestock sector is a dominant source of world food economy and apart from their social, cultural and economic role; livestock food products also act as a source of complete protein and thus, help to maintain the balanced nutrition.

Increasing temperature may result in severe economic losses and may emerge as one of the major issues for farmers all over the world. Elevated temperature not only affects animal welfare but also impacts their economic returns. Economic losses can result from reduced growth rate, meat, milk and egg production, semen quality, reproductive disorders and increasing mortality rates (Dittrich et al., 2017).

Heat stress caused an annual cost between $1.69 and $2.36 billion in US livestock industries, and out of that around 40–60% costs arising from dairy sector alone (Key and Sneeringer, 2014). Heat stress also was found to cause economic losses to the tune of 2.4 billion dollars in US livestock sector, including dairy cattle, beef cattle, swine and poultry (Nejad et al., 2015). About 25% of reduction in animal productivity is expected due to prolonged heat stress exposures and this projected reduction in production as a result of reduced growth, meat and milk production and reproduction may cause severe economic burden for the poor and marginal farmers (Rojas-Downing et al., 2017).

Elevated temperature may cause a significant economic burden to dairy industry, and the loss was estimated to be $900 million per year (Baumgard and Rhoads, 2013). Further, the heat wave caused more than 1 billion dollars of economic burden to the Californian dairy farmers (Collier et al., 2007). An economic impact study of heat stress projected a loss of about $39,000 in an average dairy, which all together contribute 1.2 billion dollars annual production loss in the United States alone (Key and Sneeringer, 2014). A recent study projected the economic loss of $49.1 and $125.8 million/year by 2050 and 2100, respectively in US dairy industry and they attributed this loss primarily to the reduced DMI in these animals (Hristov et al., 2018).

5. Pathways Associated with HS in Livestock

The neuroendocrine pathways play a key role in regulation of heat stress in livestock. There are two main neuro-endocrine adaptive mechanisms shown by the animals in response to heat stress which includes SAM and the HPA axes. These two axes function concordantly and synergistically.

The endocrinal mechanism during heat stress is controlled by HPA axis. It is comprised of CRH neurons in the hypothalamus, corticotrophs in the anterior pituitary and the adrenal cortex. In response to the stimuli the paraventricular nucleus in the hypothalamus get stimulated resulting in the secretion of CRH and vasopressin. The stimulation by CRH results in the secretion of ACTH by the corticotrophs in the anterior pituitary which in turn acts on the adrenal cortex and secretes Glucocorticoids. ACTH and glucocorticoids ultimately control the stress response pathways in animals (Afsal et al., 2018).

The SAM axis functions concurrently or often prior to stimulation of HPA axis. The exposure to heat stress results in the release of epinephrine and nor-epinephrine from the adrenal medulla and peripheral sympathetic nerves respectively. The sympathetic nervous system regulates many functions in the body including the cardiovascular, gastrointestinal, respiratory and renal systems, all of which can be modulated in response to SMS activation. The increased epinephrine concentration in the brain alarms the animal for adaptive process like decreased feed intake and HPA axis activation (Burdick et al., 2011).

The cellular mechanism is a part of acute systemic response to heat stress and is mediated by alteration of gene expression coordinating the intra and extracellular signals. In animals, an evolutionarily conserved heat shock or cellular stress response is triggered during thermal stress. This is pathway is complex and involves a cascade of protein activation and expression of genes, coordinated across a wide range of cells and tissues to minimize the adverse effects of heat load on cellular functions. The duration and extent of these alterations determines the fate of the cell- survival, acclimation or cell death. There are three major responses evoked in response to heat stress; initially, expression of chaperones and heat shock genes are elevated that acts to prevent misfolding and aggregation of protein, thereby helping in cell survival; extracellular presence of HSPs triggers various immune system activation; and finally, the continued exposure to severe stress leads to expression of cell cycle arrestors, tumor suppressors, and genes involved in apoptotic processes to prevent tumorigenesis (Collier et al., 2008).

Heat stress response consists of Heat shock factor (HSF), Heat shock element (HSE), and Heat shock proteins (HSP). HSFs are the first responders during exposure to thermal stress and have the central role in coordinating heat stress response. Of the 3 isoforms of HSF identified in animals, HSF 1 and 3 are functionally stress-responsive activators and both have maximal heat shock responsiveness. The HSF 3 is found only in poultry. The HSF are found in inert monomeric form in the cell cytoplasm associated with HSPs. During heat stress the hydrophobic domain of unfolded proteins bind to HSF. This binding results in separation from HSPs and activation by hyperphosphorylation by protein kinase which is then translocated into nucleus. Trimerization occurs in the nucleus. The activated HSFs then bind to heat shock elements (HSE) which are the specific promoter region in HSP leading to enhanced transcription of mRNA (Gupta et al., 2013).

Heat shock proteins are a family of proteins helps in cell survival during heat stress and are widely present in all species of animals. They act as molecular chaperones helping in the assembly of protein in its native conformation without being part of it (Ellis, 1987). Thus during heat stress, cellular homeostasis is maintained by HSPs. HSP 110, 90, 70, 60 and 27 are the major heat shock proteins found in the mammalian cells. HSP 70 is the most abundant and important in protection of the cells during heat stress and is considered as the golden marker for indicating heat stress in animals (Archana et al., 2017).

Heat stress is associated with compromised immune system and has adverse effect on animal health. The presence of extracellular HSPs triggers various immune cell activation (Srikanth et al., 2017) increasing the expression of Toll-like receptors (TLRs) during heat stress. The innate and adaptive immunity of the animal is activated by TLR signaling pathways. In males, mitogen-activated protein kinase (MAPK) signaling pathway is involved in reduced fertility from sperm damage due to heat stress (Rahman et al., 2014).

Although the activation of HSF in response to thermal stress protects the cell from apoptosis, the failure to activate and maintain the protective response due to intense stress results in the activation of signaling cascades that ultimately results in cell death pathways. Together with cell cycle arrest this is a protective mechanism by which tumorigenesis is arrested (Li et al., 2012). Heat stress leads to cell anomaly and DNA damage which leads to the expression of the tumor suppressors, the cell cycle arrestors, along with the activation of genes involved in apoptosis. P53 mediated cell signaling pathways are involved in apoptosis related to heat stress.

6. Pathways Associated with Adrenal Gland for HS Relief in Livestock

Adaptation of livestock to heat stress includes complex pathways involving various organs forming multiple axes like HPA, somatotrophic axis, lactotrophic axis, gonadotrophic axis and thyrotrophic axis. However, the most consistent and spontaneous response to heat stress is via the activation of the HPA axis (Binsiya et al., 2017). The signals of stress, during changing climatic conditions, are transmitted to the paraventricular nucleus (PVN) of hypothalamus by the peripheral nervous system. These stimulate the hypophysiotropic neurons to release the principle regulator of HPA axis, CRF. The CRF released into the hypophysial portal vessels target the anterior pituitary gland which then secretes the ACTH and releases it into the systemic circulation. The principal target of ACTH is the adrenal cortex thereby leading to the synthesis and secretion of glucocorticoids from the zona fasciculata (Madhusoodan et al., 2019). Glucocorticoids are the final products of the HPA axis which elicits various metabolisms and behavioral responses in heat stressed animals.

Along with the CRF, vasopressin (VP) also plays a crucial role in stimulating ACTH during heat stress. The involvement of CRF is mainly observed during the acute phase of stress while VP exerts its potential influence on the HPA axis during chronic heat stress wherein the animals are exposes to the stressful conditions repeatedly (Binsiya et al., 2017). Apart from this, pro-inflammatory cytokines like interleukin-1, interleukin-6 and tumor necrosis factor also stimulate the stress axis. However, these cytokines exert an inhibitory role on the HPA axis by stimulating the secretion of the hormone leptin from the adipocytes (Sejian, 2013). Additionally, melatonin, released from the pineal gland, have been stated to have receptors on the adrenal cortex binding to which leads to an inhibition of the ACTH stimulated cortisol production in heat stressed goats (Sejian and Srivastava 2010).

The adrenal gland is the final point in the HPA axis pathway releasing the glucocorticoids into the blood stream. Cortisol, the principle glucocorticoid, is transported through the circulatory system by the carrier protein albumin. Glucocorticoids exert a catabolic, anti-reproductive and immunosuppressive effect so as to maintain homeostasis in heat stressed animals (Tsigos et al., 2002). The physiological effects of glucocorticoids are mediated by the glucocorticoid receptors (GRs) which are widely distributed throughout the brain and peripheral tissues. During the inactive stage, GR exists as a multiprotein complex in the cytoplasm of most cells. Binding to the hormone induces conformational changes in the GR which then binds to the glucocorticoid response elements (GREs) in promoter region of glucocorticoid responsive genes thereby regulating target gene expression either positively or negatively. The GR could also regulate activation of target genes through protein-protein interaction with transcription factors apart from GRE binding (Smith and Vale, 2006).

Another secretion from the adrenal gland alleviating heat stress in livestock is aldosterone. This hormone is secreted by the zona glomerulosa of the adrenal cortex. Heat stressed animals experience severe dehydration, mainly due to the evaporative losses by the body to cope up to the thermal load. The reduction in the blood flow in the kidney activates the renin-angiotensin-aldosterone pathway. Aldosterone elicits the reabsorption of water and ions from the kidney thereby avoiding electrolyte loss and maintaining homeostasis (Afsal et al., 2018).

Though the release of glucocorticoids by the adrenal cortex aids in heat stress amelioration however, its prolonged release would be deleterious to the animal. This condition is avoided by the negative inhibition of the HPA axis by the circulating glucocorticoids. This is regulated by the binding of the glucocorticoids to the GRs located in the brain. These GRs are expressed in hypophysiotropic neurons of the PVN and thus it is considered to be the primary site for the glucocorticoid inhibition on the HPA axis. The hippocampus, containing both the GR and mineralo-corticoid receptors (MRs), is the secondary site for the negative feedback on the axis. Glucocorticoids have a low nanomolar affinity for GRs and extensively bind to them during elevated periods of glucocorticoid secretion that occur following stress. Though the MRs has subnanomolar affinity for glucocorticoids, they have a restricted expression pattern in the brain to glucocorticoids during basal secretion. Therefore, the MRs regulates the basal HPA tone and the GRs mediate negative feedback mechanism following stress (Smith and Vale, 2006).

7. Products of Adrenal Gland for Regulation of HEAT Stress in Livestock

Neuro-endocrine regulation acts as a potent adaptive mechanism which enables the animal to cope up to heat stress. Adrenal gland being an integral part of the HPA and SAM axis plays a pivotal role during heat stress. Glucocorticoids and aldosterone, secreted from the adrenal cortex and catecholamines, secreted from the adrenal medulla are the primary endocrine regulators during heat stress. Cortisol, the primary glucocorticoid, acts on various tissues thereby initiating a number of mechanisms and biochemical processes which helps to maintain homeostasis. During heat stress, animals are subjected to severe dehydration which plays a crucial role to maintain the fluid and electrolyte homeostasis in the body. Catecholamines mainly including dopamine, adrenaline and noradrenaline, integrates certain adaptive responses in animals during stress. They also play a chief role in regulating various physiological responses thereby enabling animals to adapt during heat stress (Binsiya et al., 2017; Afsal et al., 2018).

8. Functions of Adrenal Gland during Heat Stress in Livestock

Adrenal gland plays a very crucial role in controlling heat stress in animals. These are paired glands located above each kidney and hence also known as suprarenal glands. The gland is divided into cortex and medulla and their secretions have distinct functions. The adrenal cortex is divided into three distinct zones. The outer zone is the zona glomerulosa which produces the steroid hormone aldosterone. Greater than 70% of the cortex comprises zona fasciculata. The secretory cells of this layer produce glucocorticoids. The inner most layer is the zona reticularis produces small amounts of sex steroids androgens, estrogens and progestins in some species (Rosol et al., 2001).

Adrenal gland is an intricate part of neuroendocrine pathways which helps the animal to adapt to the stressful conditions. These pathways include hypothalamus-pituitary-adrenal (HPA) axis and sympathetic-adrenal-medullary (SAM). The hypothalamus-pituitary-adrenal (HPA) axis is the primary neuroendocrine system involved in the stress response. Glucocorticoids from adrenal cortex are the primary product from HPA axis activation while catecholamines from adrenal medulla are the secretory products from SAM axis activation. Both these axis play a crucial role in stress relieving in animals.

Acute heat stress is always associated with marked elevations in the level of glucocorticoids, especially cortisol which is the main glucocorticoid hormone and hence it is regarded as the golden marker for heat stress response in animals. Cortisol is a steroid hormone synthesized from cholesterol and is transported in blood by cortisol binding globulin (CBG). A small portion of the hormone circulates in free form. Following a heat exposure the animal responds immediately by the increased secretion of cortisol. The concentration of glucocorticoids increases initially from a level of 2.4 μg/100 ml to 3.9 μg/100 ml (62%) attains a peak level of 5.4 μg/100 ml (120%). The level then declines gradually to normal concentration in spite of the continuing heat stimulus as the animal gradually readjust into thermo neutrality (Alvarez and Johnson, 1973). The release of cortisol is under the influence of ACTH from the anterior pituitary. The increased secretion of ACTH and consequent increase in the level of glucocorticoids are critical for successful adaptation of the animal to thrive over extreme environmental temperature. Glucocorticoids are regarded as an integrating signal which in combination with other endocrine secretions determines the behavioral, physiological and metabolic changes which helps the animal to adapt to the harsh stressful conditions (Sejian et al., 2010).

The major function of cortisol is the stimulation of hepatic gluconeogenesis which converts non-carbohydrates sources into glucose. Heat stressed animals are under a state of negative energy balance from reduced feed intake and reduced metabolism. The energy available will be diverted for maintaining homeostasis by the animal. The cortisol plays a major role by mobilization of energy to meet the energy requirements of the vital organs. It stimulates glycogenolysis, lipolysis and proteolysis in heat stressed animal.

Cortisol also functions as vasodilators and helps the animal to dissipate more heat to the environment by increasing the peripheral blood flow (Farooq et al., 2010).

Plasma cortisol decreases the available quantities of the calorigenic hormone like thyroid hormones and growth hormone. Cortisol decreases the concentration of T3 by inhibiting the biotransformation of T4 to T3 (Lenis et al., 2016). This is an adaptive mechanism by the animal to decrease the heat load by decreasing the metabolic heat from the body. The endogenous heat load is thus reduced and the animal brought into thermal balance with its environment (Christison & Johnson, 1972).

Although glucocorticoids has a beneficiary role in maintaining homeostasis, the prolonged stimulation of the HPA axis and resulting increase in the glucocorticoids has a negative impact on the animal health by suppression of immune function and reproductive efficiency (Afsal et al., 2018).

Aldosterone is another important hormone secreted from the adrenal cortex and plays a major role in maintaining fluid and electrolyte homeostasis in the body during heat stress. High environmental temperatures results in increased secretion of aldosterone, which is a part of Renin-Angiotensin-Aldosterone system. During periods of heat stress there will be increased water loss from the body via skin and respiratory evaporation as a part of behavioral response to dissipate body heat (Bernabucci et al., 2010). This may cause disturbance in fluid and mineral balance in the body. Hypovolemia resulting from severe dehydration during heat stress causes the juxtaglomerular apparatus in the kidney to secrete renin. This hormone stimulates the synthesis of angiotensin which in turn results in the secretion of aldosterone from adrenal cortex. The major site of action of aldosterone is on the distal tubules and collecting ducts of the kidney. Aldosterone maintains the vascular pressure by reabsorbing water and ions, mainly sodium ions thus minimizing the excretion of water (Bhimte et al., 2018).

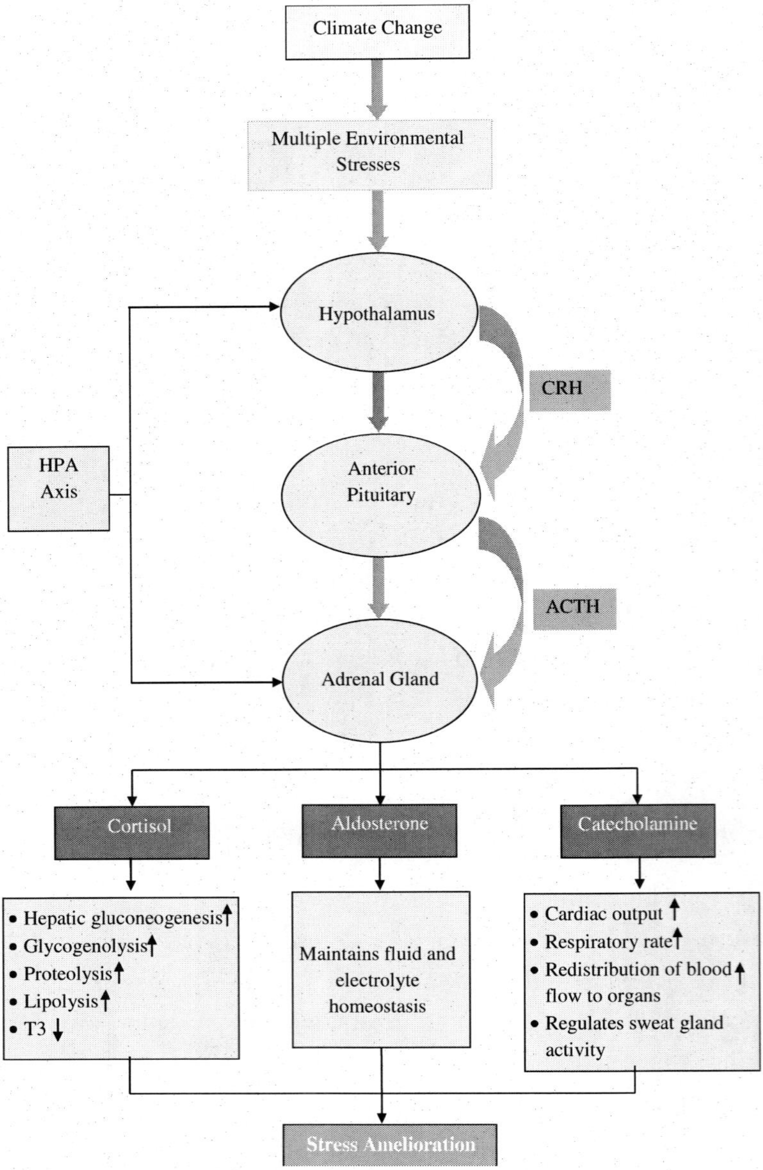

Figure 1. Role of adrenal gland in heat stress amelioration in farm animals. The figure describes the mechanism by which heat stress activates HPA axis and how the endocrine products of adrenal gland elicit different adaptive mechanisms to maintain homeostasis in farm animals. HPA– Hypothalamus-Pituitary-Adrenal axis; T3 – Tri-Iodo-Thyronine.

Activation of the sympathetic adrenal medullary (SAM) axis and associated receptors occurs rapidly on exposure to stressful condition resulting in the secretion of the catecholamines - adrenaline and noradrenaline. Epinephrine is secreted from adrenal medulla while nor-epinephrine from peripheral sympathetic nerves and are circulated through blood. Catecholamines concentration increases during both acute and chronic heat stress. The ratio of epinephrine to norepinephrine secreted varies depending on the species of the animals. In most of the animals including cattle, epinephrine is the major hormone secreted from adrenal medulla (Burdick et al., 2011). During periods of heat stress, the concentration of epinephrine and nor-epinephrine respectively increases by 45 and 42% in short and 91 and 70% in long term heat exposure (Alvarez and Johnson, 1973). These hormones play an important role in integrating adaptive mechanism during stress, especially flight and fright responses. Catecholamines increases cardiac output, respiratory rate and redistribution of blood flow to pulmonary organs and other organs which are necessary for increasing heat responses. In cattle, catecholamines also regulate the activity of sweat glands (Farooq et al., 2010). Figure 1 describes the mechanisms by which heat stress triggers activation of HPA axis to relieve heat stress in farm animals.

9. Glucocorticoids Action on Various Tissues in Livestock during Heat Stress

The physiological and reproductive statuses of the animals are very much influenced by the environmental temperature. Heat stress evokes coordination of behavioral, physiological and neuroendocrine regulation for adaptation to heat stress maintaining homeostatis. One of the key regulators of heat stress adaptation is by the endocrine system.

Glucocorticoids are steroid hormones secreted by adrenal cortex by the activation of HPA axis. The HPA axis activation is the central and complex adaptive response to heat stress. HPA axis is comprised of CRH neurons in the hypothalamus, corticotrophs in the anterior pituitary and the adrenal cortex. The external stimuli from the skin receptors reach the hypothalamus which secretes ACTH which finally acts on the adrenal cortex in secreting glucocorticoids to exert its function in target tissues mainly liver, muscle and adipose tissue. The most important response to heat stress in animals is the secretion of cortisol. Glucocorticoids can affect the concentration of non-esterified fatty acids, lactate, plasma insulin and although having a variable effect on glucose metabolism (Afsal et al., 2018). Majority of cortisol is carried by plasma albumin. Transcortin, a cortisol binding globulin also carries cortisol while 1-10% exists in free form. Large quantities of cortisol are secreted by cows in response to acute heat stress than chronic heat stress (Christison and Johnson, 1972). Glucocorticoid levels continue to decline gradually as the animal acclimates to a chronic, mild heat exposure.

Cortisol, also known as hydrocortisone contributes to about 95 per cent of glucocorticoid activity of the adrenocortical secretion. Large quantities of cortisol are secreted by the animals in response to acute heat stress. Plasma cortisol levels remains elevated for about 12 hours after the initial exposure to extreme temperature and decreases to normal levels within 2 days while the animals readjusts to thermo-neutrality (Christison and Johnson, 1972). During heat stress cortisol acts by mobilization of energy for maintenance of muscular and neural functions, directly influencing metabolism and behavior of animals exposed to thermal stress. Cortisol restores the homeostasis of the heat stressed animal by stimulating glycogenolysis, lipolysis and proteolysis.

Cortisol and other glucocorticoids have an overall anabolic effect in liver tissue during heat stress. One of the major actions of glucocorticoids under heat stress is the amplified rate of hepatic gluconeogenesis, resulting in an increased level of endogenous glucose from non-carbohydrate sources. This ensure the supply of glucose to extrahepatic targets like brain, erythrocytes and renal medulla compensating heat stress induced hypoglycemic condition from reduced feed intake.

Cortisol enters and binds to the glucocorticoid receptor in the cytoplasm of the hepatocytes. This hormone-receptor complex then enters the cell nucleus to activate DNA transcription with formation of mRNA which ultimately leads to the synthesis of enzymes required for gluconeogenesis. The gene expression of pyruvate carboxylase, a rate limiting in gluconeogenesis pathway which converts pyruvate to oxaloacetate making the entry of lactate and alanine in gluconeogenic pathway is increased in different animal models studied under heat stress. Main regulatory enzymes are pyruvate carboxylase (PC), which converts pyruvate into oxaloacetate, phosphoenolpyruvate carboxykinase (PEPCK) promoting the decarboxylation of oxaloacetate to phosphoenolpyruvate, and finally glucose- 6-phosphatase (G6Pase), hydrolysing glucose-6-phosphate into free glucose and inorganic phosphate (Rhoads et al., 2013b).

Hepatic glycogenolysis also contributes to increased hepatic glucose output during thermal stress. Glucocorticoids also increase the uptake of amino acids by hepatic cells thereby enhancing gluconeogenesis in the liver. Synthesis of proteins also occurs in the liver thus increasing the total hepatic protein output. Increased rate of gluconeogenesis leads to marked increase of glycogen in the hepatocytes. This may lead to the action of other glycolytic hormones such as epinephrine and glucagon, to mobilize glucose in times of need.

Glucocorticoids inhibit the synthesis or secretion of Corticotrophin releasing hormone (CRH), vasopressin and ACTH, thus exerting a negative feedback mechanism on hypothalamus and pituitary.

One of the immediate effects of glucocorticoids during heat stress is vasodilatation. This helps the animal in dissipating more heat to the environment (Farooq et al., 2010). In skeletal muscle glucocorticoids have a catabolic effect during heat stress. The skeletal muscle being the major store of amino acids, the proteolytic action of glucocorticoids on skeletal muscle increases the level of free amino acids. These amino acids provide substrate for hepatic gluconeogenesis (Sejian et al., 2008).

The reproductive efficiency and overall fertility of the animals is compromised during heat stress. Glucocorticoids are required for proper gonadal function and are controlled at the hypothalamo-pituitary-gonadal axis. The ACTH stimulated glucocorticoids released in association with heat stress mediates an inhibitory action on reproduction induced by heat stress. Glucocorticoids inhibit meiotic maturation of oocytes, follicular development and ovulation by follicular selection and dominance (Krishnan et al., 2017). Glucocorticoids also reduce the fertility in male by directly acting on the testis. Elevated levels of this hormone declines the level of testosterone, thereby affecting spermatogenesis, libido and thus the overall fertility in animals.

Glucocorticoids also have effects in the secretion of other endocrine hormones. It affects the thyroid gland by decreasing the concentration of T3 by inhibiting the biotransformation of T4 to T3 (Lenis et al., 2016).

Many of the immune cells possess glucocorticoid receptors. Binding of cortisol to the receptor in response to heat stress interfere with the function of NF-kB cytokine expression and has been reported to lead to immunosupression and increased susceptibility to antigenic challenge in different animals. (Padgett & Glaser, 2003).

The secretion of preformed Heat Shock Proteins (HSPs) is under the control of glucocorticoids. The preformed HSPs are bound to glucocorticoid receptor in the cell cytoplasm. Binding of the hormone releases the receptor bound proteins helping in protecting protein structure thus forming the first line of defense during heat stress (Rhoads et al., 2009).

Another interesting fact about glucocorticoids is that they can bind to both glucocorticoid receptor and mineralocorticoid receptor, possessing more affinity for the latter. Unlike glucocorticoid receptors which are ubiquitously found in the body, receptors for mineralocorticoids are found in hippocampus, heart, kidney and colon. In addition to this, glucocorticoids can modulate the expression of the β-adrenergic receptor both through genomic and nongenomic means. Thus together with catecholamines, glucocorticoids increase cardiac output (Burdick et al., 2011).

10. Regulators of Adrenal Gland and of HPA Axis

The neuro-endocrine regulation during heat stress is considered as the principal adaptive mechanism exhibited by animals and among them, the HPA axis play an integral role. Stressors like heat stress, drought, nutritional stress and/or disease activates the HPA axis. These stimuli are transmitted by the sense organs which on coordination by the brain center activates the HPA axis (Afsal et al., 2018).

The rise in environmental temperature due to rapidly changing climatic conditions leads to the release of CRF, the principal regulator of the HPA axis, and arginine-vasopressin (AVP) in livestock (Sejian et al., 2010). The release of CRF initiates a cascade of events which finally acts on the adrenal cortex leading to the secretion of the end product of the axis, the glucocorticoids. The glucocorticoids exert physiological and behavioral effects on heat stressed animals enabling them to maintain homeostasis. The endocrine action of adreno-corticotrophic hormone (ACTH), CRH and AVP mediate glucocorticoid secretion from the adrenal cortex. Based on the impact and duration of stress, the release of glucocorticoids are managed which also regulates the HPA axis by exerting a negative feedback (Binsiya et al., 2017).

Apart from heat stress, nutritional stress also regulates the HPA axis followed by secretions from the adrenal gland. Sejian et al. (2010) reported increased cortisol levels in Malpura rams which were subjected to a combination of heat and nutritional stress. Severe impact on biological functions were observed in sheep subjected to combined stress which resulted in an increased cortisol secretion from the adrenal gland when compared to that during heat stress or nutritional stress alone. This highlights that based on the severity of stress the secretions of HPA axis and adrenal gland are regulated.

Another stressor having a regulatory role on HPA axis is aggressive behavior. Aggression and glucocorticoid levels share a negative correlation in many species including pigs and cattle (Curley Jr. et al., 2008; Muráni et al., 2010). The regulatory effects of aggressive behavior on adrenal gland and HPA axis show variations among individual which have been attributed due to genetic factors. Nucleotide sequence variations and QTLs in genes like *Corticosteroid binding globulin encoding* (*CBG*) and *Ryanodine receptor 1* (*RYR1*) have been stated to affect basal functioning of the HPA axis and cortisol levels. Also at the molecular level, genes encoding the various members of the HPA axis pathway (*CRH* (corticotropin-releasing hormone), *CRHR1* (CRH type 1 receptor), *CRHBP* (CRH binding protein), *AVP* (vasopressin), *AVPR1B* (vasopressin V1B receptor), *POMC* (proopiomelanocortin), *MC2R* (melanocortin type 2 (ACTH) receptor), *NR3C1* (glucocorticoid receptor)) and the CRH members (*UCN* (urocortin), *CRHR2* (CRH type 2 receptor)) also play an influential role in the regulation and modulation of HPA axis and adrenal gland (Steckler, 2001; Muráni et al., 2010).

CONCLUSION

Heat stress acts as the major detrimental factor for livestock production. Therefore, understanding the underlying biological mechanisms by which the animals cope with heat stress is very essential. This particular chapter highlights the role of adrenal gland in relieving heat stress in domestic livestock species. The chapter describes in detail the pathways associated with both heat stress as well as the pathways associated with HPA axis to relieve heat stress in livestock. The adrenal gland through its secretions both from adrenal cortex and adrenal medulla counters the heat stress. The adrenal cortex through its primary secretion of glucocorticoids helps the animals to survive the heat stress. The primary role of glucocorticoid is to maintain energy balance to support the life sustaining activities. Further, through the secretion of aldosterone, adrenal cortex plays a significant role in maintaining the electrolyte balance. In addition through the secretions of catecholamines from the adrenal medulla, adrenal gland controls the physiological variables by increasing the blood supply to maintain pulmonary functions to dissipate body heat. Overall, the chapter provides a detailed description of role of adrenal gland during heat stress and the different functions of this particular endocrine gland to maintain homeostasis in animals.

FUTURE PERSPECTIVES

Given the significance of livestock to meet the global food demand of the future it becomes increasingly essential to sustain livestock production in the changing climate scenario. As heat stress seems to be the major intriguing factor reducing the economy of livestock farms, it is very essential to identify ways and means to cope the livestock production system to this particular environmental stress. Scientific communities are battling in its efforts to identify different biological markers to quantify heat stress response in farm animals in an effort to develop suitable amelioration strategies to sustain their production. Although there are few confirmatory biological markers identified for heat stress impact on livestock production, farming community needs several other important biomarkers to quantify heat stress response. This will help in finding the grass root solution for the heat stress associated production loss in farm animals. Further, detailed research are needed to elucidate the pathways associated with heat stress in affecting livestock production as well on the pathways of HPA axis in an effort to identify new ways to target reducing the adverse impacts of heat stress on livestock production. Such efforts should be multi disciplinary to ensure appropriate productive and reproductive ability to these animals, in addition to imparting them the efficiency to survive in different agro-ecological zones.

REFERENCES

Afsal, A. V, Sejian, M., Bagath, G., Krishnan, C., Devaraj and R., Bhatta. "Heat stress and livestock adaptation: Neuro-endocrine regulation."

International Journal of Veterinary and Animal Medicine 1, no. 2 (2018): 1-8. https://doi.org/10.31021/ijvam.20181108.

Archana, Payyanakkal Ravindranathan, Joy, Aleena, Prathap, Pragna, Mallenahally Kusha, Vidya, P. A. A., Niyas, Madiajagan, Bagath, and Govindan, Krishnan et al. "Role of Heat Shock Proteins in Livestock Adaptation to Heat Stress." *Journal of Dairy, Veterinary & Animal Research* 5, no. 1 (2017): 13–19. https://doi.org/10.15406/jdvar.2017.05.00127.

Baumgard, Lance H., and Robert P. Rhoads. "Effects of Heat Stress on Postabsorptive Metabolism and Energetics." *Annual review of animal biosciences* 1 (2013): 311–37. https://doi.org/10.1146/annurev-animal-031412-103644.

Baumgard, Lance H., Robert P. Rhoads, Michelle L. Rhoads, Nicholas K. Gabler, Jason W. Ross, Aileen F. Keating, Rebbeca L. Boddicker, Sangeeta Lenka, and Veerasamy Sejian. "Impact of Climate Change on Livestock Production." In *Environmental Stress and Amelioration in Livestock Production*. Edited by Veerasamy Sejian et al., 413–68. Berlin, Heidelberg: Springer Berlin Heidelberg, 2012. https://doi.org/10.1007/978-3-642-29205-7_15.

Bernabucci, U., L. Basiricò, and P. Morera. "Impact of Hot Environment on Colostrum and Milk Composition." *Cellular and molecular biology (Noisy-le-Grand, France)* 59, no. 1 (2013): 67–83.

Binsiya TK, Sejian V, Bagath M, Krishnan G, Hyder I, Manimaran A, Lees AM, Gaughan JB, Bhatta R. "Significance of hypothalamic-pituitary-adrenal axis to adapt to climate change in livestock." *International Research Journal of Agricultural and Food Sciences* 2 (2017): 1–20.

Burdick, N. C., R. D. Randel, J. A. Carroll, and T. H. Welsh. "Interactions Between Temperament, Stress, and Immune Function in Cattle." *International Journal of Zoology* 2011 (2011):1-9. https://doi.org/10.1155/2011/373197.

Chauhan, S. S., P. Celi, B. J. Leury, I. J. Clarke, and F. R. Dunshea. "Dietary Antioxidants at Supranutritional Doses Improve Oxidative Status and Reduce the Negative Effects of Heat Stress in Sheep."

Journal of animal science 92, no. 8 (2014): 3364–74. https://doi.org/10.2527/jas.2014-7714.

Christison, G. I., and H. D. Johnson. "Cortisol Turnover in Heat-Stressed Cow." *Journal of animal science* 35, no. 5 (1972): 1005–10. https://doi.org/10.2527/jas1972.3551005x.

Collier, J. L., M. B. Abdallah, L. L. Hernandez, J. V. Norgaard, and R. J. Collier. "Prostaglandins A1 (PGA1) and E1 (PGE1) Alter Heat Chock Protein 70 (HSP-70) Gene Expression in Bovine Mammary Epithelial Cells (BMEC)." *Journal of animal science*, Suppl. 1 (2007).

Collier, R. J., J. L. Collier, R. P. Rhoads, and L. H. Baumgard. "Invited Review: Genes Involved in the Bovine Heat Stress Response." *Journal of dairy science* 91, no. 2 (2008): 445–54. https://doi.org/10.3168/jds.2007-0540.

Cunningham J. C. and Klein B. G. "Endocrinology" In *Textbook of veterinary physiology* 4th edn. Saunders 439–448. Elsevier, St. Louis, 2007

Curley Jr., Kevin O., Don A. Neuendorff, Andrew W. Lewis, Jason J. Cleere, Thomas H. Welsh Jr, and Ronald D. Randel. "Functional Characteristics of the Bovine Hypothalamic-Pituitary-Adrenal Axis Vary with Temperament." *Hormones and behavior* 53, no. 1 (2008): 20–27. https://doi.org/10.1016/j.yhbeh.2007.08.005.

da Silva, Wilma Emanuela, Jacinara Hody Gurgel Morais Leite, José Ernandes Rufino de Sousa, Wirton Peixoto Costa, Wallace Sostene Tavares da Silva, Magda Maria Guilhermino, Luis Alberto Bermejo Asensio, and Débora Andréa Evangelista Façanha. "Daily Rhythmicity of the Thermoregulatory Responses of Locally Adapted Brazilian Sheep in a Semiarid Environment." *International Journal of Biometeorology* 61, no. 7 (2017): 1221–31. https://doi.org/10.1007/s00484-016-1300-2.

Dittrich, Ruth, Anita Wreford, Cairistiona F. E. Topp, Vera Eory, and Dominic Moran. "A Guide Towards Climate Change Adaptation in the Livestock Sector: Adaptation Options and the Role of Robust Decision-Making Tools for Their Economic Appraisal." *Regional*

Environmental Change 17, no. 6 (2017): 1701–12. https://doi.org/10.1007/s10113-017-1134-4.

Ellis, R. J. "Proteins as Molecular Chaperones." *Nature* 328, no. 6129 (1987): 378–79. https://doi.org/10.1038/328378a0.

FAO (Food and Agriculture Organization of the United Nations) *Coping with Climate Change: The Roles of Genetic Resources for Food and Agriculture*. Rome: Food and Agriculture Organization of the United Nations, 2015.

Farooq, U, H.A. Samad, F. Shehzad and A. Qayyum. "Physiological Responses of Cattle to Heat Stress." *World Applied Sciences Journal* 8, (Special Issue of Biotechnology & Genetic Engineering) (2010): 38–43.

Garkal, R. A., P. M. Kekan, S. D. Kharde, V. K. Munde, B. W. Narladkar, and M. S. Vaidya. "Effect of Different Housing Systems on Haematological Parameters of Buffaloes." *Buffalo Bulletin* 35 no. 2 (2016): 191–98. http://kuojs.lib.ku.ac.th/index.php/BufBu/article/view/1290.

Gaughan, John B., Veerasamy Sejian, Terry L. Mader, and Frank R. Dunshea. "Adaptation Strategies: Ruminants." *Animal Frontiers* 9, no. 1 (2019): 47–53. https://doi.org/10.1093/af/vfy029.

Gupta, N. K., Shubhi Agarwal, V. P. Agarwal, N. S. Nathawat, Sunita Gupta, and G. Singh. "Effect of Short-Term Heat Stress on Growth, Physiology and Antioxidative Defence System in Wheat Seedlings." *Acta Physiologiae Plantarum* 35, no. 6 (2013): 1837–42. https://doi.org/10.1007/s11738-013-1221-1.

Hristov, A. N., A. T. Degaetano, C. A. Rotz, E. Hoberg, R. H. Skinner, T. Felix, and H. Li et al. "Climate Change Effects on Livestock in the Northeast US and Strategies for Adaptation." *Climatic Change* 146, no. 1 (2018): 33–45. https://doi.org/10.1007/s10584-017-2023-z.

Key, N., and S. Sneeringer. "Potential Effects of Climate Change on the Productivity of U.S. Dairies." *American Journal of Agricultural Economics* 96, no. 4 (2014): 1136–56. https://doi.org/10.1093/ajae/aau002.

Krishnan, Govindan, Madiajagan Bagath, Prathap Pragna, Mallenahally Kusha Vidya, Joy Aleena, Payyanakkal Ravindranathan Archana, Veerasamy Sejian, and Raghavendra Bhatta. "Mitigation of the Heat Stress Impact in Livestock Reproduction." In *Theriogenology*. Edited by Rita P. Carreira. InTech, 2017.

Lenis Sanin, Yasser, Angélica María Zuluaga Cabrera, and Ariel Marcel Tarazona Morales. "Adaptive Responses to Thermal Stress in Mammals." *Revista de Medicina Veterinaria* 31 (2016): 121–35. http://www.scielo.org.co/scielo.php?script=sci_arttext&pid=S0122-93542016000100012&nrm=iso.

Li, Tongyuan, Ning Kon, Le Jiang, Minjia Tan, Thomas Ludwig, Yingming Zhao, Richard Baer, and Wei Gu. "Tumor Suppression in the Absence of P53-Mediated Cell-Cycle Arrest, Apoptosis, and Senescence." *Cell* 149, no. 6 (2012): 1269–83. https://doi.org/10.1016/j.cell.2012.04.026.

Madhusoodan, Aradotlu Parameshwarappa, Sejian Veerasamy, Rashamol Veettiparambil Pandarathil, Savitha Sira Tulasiramu, Bagath Madiajagan, Krishnan Govindan, and Bhatta Raghavendra. "Resilient Capacity of Cattle to Environmental Challenges – an Updated Review." *Journal of Animal Behaviour and Biometeorology* 7, no. 3 (2019): 104–18. https://doi.org/10.31893/2318-1265jabb.v7n3p104-118.

Mazzullo, Giuseppe, Claudia Rifici, Gino Caccamo, Maria Rizzo, and Giuseppe Piccione. "Effect of Different Environmental Conditions on Some Haematological Parameters in Cow." *Annals of Animal Science* 14, no. 4 (2014): 947–54. https://doi.org/10.2478/aoas-2014-0049.

Muráni, Eduard, Siriluck Ponsuksili, Richard B. D'Eath, Simon P. Turner, Esra Kurt, Gary Evans, and Ludger Thölking et al. "Association of HPA Axis-Related Genetic Variation with Stress Reactivity and Aggressive Behaviour in Pigs." *BMC Genetics* 11, no. 1 (2010): 74. https://doi.org/10.1186/1471-2156-11-74.
https://doi.org/10.1186/1471-2156-11-74.

Naqvi, S. M. K., V. P. Maurya, R. Gulyani, A. Joshi, and J. P. Mittal. "The Effect of Thermal Stress on Superovulatory Response and Embryo

Production in Bharat Merino Ewes." *Small Ruminant Research* 55, 1-3 (2004): 57–63. https://doi.org/10.1016/j.smallrumres.2004.02.009.

Nejad, Jalil Ghassemi, Jayant D. Lohakare, Joe W. West, Byong W. Kim, Bae H. Lee, and Kyung I. Sung. "Effects of Water Restriction Following Feeding on Nutrient Digestibilities, Milk Yield and Composition and Blood Hormones in Lactating Holstein Cows Under Heat Stress Conditions." *Italian Journal of Animal Science* 14, no. 3 (2015): 3952. https://doi.org/10.4081/ijas.2015.3952.

Padgett, David A., and Ronald Glaser. "How Stress Influences the Immune Response." *Trends in immunology* 24, no. 8 (2003): 444–48. https://doi.org/10.1016/s1471-4906(03)00173-x.

Pragna, Prathap, P. R. Archana, Joy Aleena, Veerasamy Sejian, Govindan Krishnan, Madiajagan Bagath, and A. Manimaran et al. "Heat Stress and Dairy Cow: Impact on Both Milk Yield and Composition." *International Journal of Dairy Science* 12, no. 1 (2017): 1–11. https://doi.org/10.3923/ijds.2017.1.11.

Rahman, Mohammad Bozlur, Md Mostofa Kamal, Tom Rijsselaere, Leen Vandaele, Mohammed Shamsuddin, and Ann van Soom. "Altered Chromatin Condensation of Heat-Stressed Spermatozoa Perturbs the Dynamics of DNA Methylation Reprogramming in the Paternal Genome After in Vitro Fertilisation in Cattle." *Reproduction, fertility, and development* 26, no. 8 (2014): 1107–16. https://doi.org/10.1071/RD13218.

Rhoads, M. L., R. P. Rhoads, M. J. VanBaale, R. J. Collier, S. R. Sanders, W. J. Weber, B. A. Crooker, and L. H. Baumgard. "Effects of Heat Stress and Plane of Nutrition on Lactating Holstein Cows: I. Production, Metabolism, and Aspects of Circulating Somatotropin." *Journal of dairy science* 92, no. 5 (2009): 1986–97. https://doi.org/10.3168/jds.2008-1641.

Rhoads, Robert P., Lance H. Baumgard, Jessica K. Suagee, and Sara R. Sanders. "Nutritional Interventions to Alleviate the Negative Consequences of Heat Stress." *Advances in nutrition (Bethesda, Md.)* 4, no. 3 (2013a): 267–76. https://doi.org/10.3945/an.112.003376.

Rhoads, R. P., L. H. Baumgard, and J. K. Suagee. "2011 and 2012 Early Careers Achievement Awards: Metabolic Priorities During Heat Stress with an Emphasis on Skeletal Muscle1,2." *Journal of animal science* 91, no. 6 (2013b): 2492–2503. https://doi.org/10.2527/jas.2012-6120.

Ribeiro, Maria N., Neila L. Ribeiro, Riccardo Bozzi, and Roberto G. Costa. "Physiological and Biochemical Blood Variables of Goats Subjected to Heat Stress – a Review." *Journal of Applied Animal Research* 46, no. 1 (2018): 1036–41. https://doi.org/10.1080/09712119.2018.1456439.

Rojas-Downing, M. Melissa, A. Pouyan Nejadhashemi, Timothy Harrigan, and Sean A. Woznicki. "Climate Change and Livestock: Impacts, Adaptation, and Mitigation." *Climate Risk Management* 16 (2017): 145–63. https://doi.org/10.1016/j.crm.2017.02.001.

Sejian, V., R. S. Srivastava, and V. P. Varshney. "Pineal-Adrenal Relationship: Modulating Effects of Glucocorticoids on Pineal Function to Ameliorate Thermal-Stress in Goats." *Asian-Australasian Journal of Animal Sciences* 21, no. 7 (2008): 988–94. https://doi.org/10.5713/ajas.2008.70482.

Sejian, Veerasamy, and Rajendra Swaroop Srivastava. "Effects of Melatonin on Adrenal Cortical Functions of Indian Goats Under Thermal Stress." *Veterinary Medicine International* 2010, 1-2 (2010): 1–6. https://doi.org/10.4061/2010/348919.

Sejian, Veerasamy, Vijai P. Maurya, and Sayeed M. K. Naqvi. "Adaptive Capability as Indicated by Endocrine and Biochemical Responses of Malpura Ewes Subjected to Combined Stresses (Thermal and Nutritional) in a Semi-Arid Tropical Environment." *International journal of biometeorology* 54, no. 6 (2010): 653–61. https://doi.org/10.1007/s00484-010-0341-1.

Sejian, V., V. P. Maurya, and S. M. K. Naqvi. "Effect of Thermal Stress, Restricted Feeding and Combined Stresses (Thermal Stress and Restricted Feeding) on Growth and Plasma Reproductive Hormone Levels of Malpura Ewes Under Semi-Arid Tropical Environment." *Journal of animal physiology and animal nutrition* 95, no. 2 (2011): 252–58. https://doi.org/10.1111/j.1439-0396.2010.01048.x.

Sejian, Veerasamy, Vijai Prakash Maurya, Kamal Kumar, and Syed Mohammad Khursheed Naqvi. "Effect of Multiple Stresses (Thermal, Nutritional, and Walking Stress) on the Reproductive Performance of Malpura Ewes." *Veterinary Medicine International* 2012 (2012). https://doi.org/10.1155/2012/471760. http://dx.doi.org/10.1155/2012/471760.

Sejian V. "Climate Change: impact on production and reproduction, adaptation mechanisms and mitigation strategies in small ruminants: A review". *Indian Journal of Small Ruminants* 19, no.1 (2013): 1–21.

Sejian, Veerasamy, Raghavendra Bhatta, N. M. Soren, P. K. Malik, J. P. Ravindra, Cadaba S. Prasad, and Rattan Lal. "Introduction to Concepts of Climate Change Impact on Livestock and Its Adaptation and Mitigation." In *Climate Change Impact on Livestock: Adaptation and Mitigation.* Vol. 60. Edited by Veerasamy Sejian et al., 1–23. New Delhi: Springer India, 2015.

Sejian, Veerasamy, Gaughan, J. B., Bhatta, R., and Naqvi, S. M. "Impact of climate change on livestock productivity" *Feedipedia-Animal Feed Resources Information System-INRA CIRAD AFZ and FAO* (2016): 1-4

Sejian, Veerasamy, Davendra Kumar, John B. Gaughan, and Syed M.K. Naqvi. "Effect of Multiple Environmental Stressors on the Adaptive Capability of Malpura Rams Based on Physiological Responses in a Semi-Arid Tropical Environment." *Journal of Veterinary Behavior* 17 (2017): 6–13. https://doi.org/10.1016/j.jveb.2016.10.009.

Shaji, Shilja, V. Sejian, M. Bagath, G. B. Manjunathareddy, E. K. Kurien, Girish Varma, and Raghavendra Bhatta. "Summer Season Related Heat and Nutritional Stresses on the Adaptive Capability of Goats Based on Blood Biochemical Response and Hepatic HSP70 Gene Expression." *Biological Rhythm Research* 48, no. 1 (2017): 65–83. https://doi.org/10.1080/09291016.2016.1232340.

Skibiel, Amy L., Maya Zachut, Bruno C. do Amaral, Yishai Levin, and Geoffrey E. Dahl. "Liver Proteomic Analysis of Postpartum Holstein Cows Exposed to Heat Stress or Cooling Conditions During the Dry

Period." *Journal of dairy science* 101, no. 1 (2018): 705–16. https://doi.org/10.3168/jds.2017-13258.

Smith, Sean M., and Wylie W. Vale. "The Role of the Hypothalamic-Pituitary-Adrenal Axis in Neuroendocrine Responses to Stress." *Dialogues in clinical neuroscience* 8, no. 4 (2006): 383–95.

Srikanth, Krishnamoorthy, Anam Kwon, Eunjin Lee, and Hoyoung Chung. "Characterization of Genes and Pathways That Respond to Heat Stress in Holstein Calves Through Transcriptome Analysis." *Cell stress & chaperones* 22, no. 1 (2017): 29–42. https://doi.org/10.1007/s12192-016-0739-8.

Steckler, T. "The Molecular Neurobiology of Stress--Evidence from Genetic and Epigenetic Models." *Behavioural pharmacology* 12, 6-7 (2001): 381–427. https://doi.org/10.1097/00008877-200111000-00002.

Thornton, Philip K., and Pierre J. Gerber. "Climate Change and the Growth of the Livestock Sector in Developing Countries." *Mitigation and Adaptation Strategies for Global Change* 15, no. 2 (2010): 169–84. https://doi.org/10.1007/s11027-009-9210-9.

Tsigos, Constantine, and George P. Chrousos. "Hypothalamic–pituitary–adrenal Axis, Neuroendocrine Factors and Stress." *Journal of Psychosomatic Research* 53, no. 4 (2002): 865–71. https://doi.org/10.1016/S0022-3999(02)00429-4.

INDEX

D

E

F

G

H

N

O

P

T

U

V

W

Y